Introduction to Telemedicine

Second edition

Edited by

Richard Wootton, John Craig
and Victor Patterson

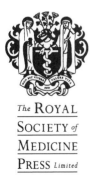

The ROYAL
SOCIETY *of*
MEDICINE
PRESS *Limited*

© 2006 Royal Society of Medicine Press Ltd

Published by the Royal Society of Medicine Press Ltd
1 Wimpole Street, London W1G 0AE, UK
Tel: +44 (0)20 7290 2921
Fax: +44 (0)20 7290 2929
Email: publishing@rsm.ac.uk
Website: www.rsmpress.co.uk

British Library Cataloguing in Publication Data
A catalogue record for this book is available from the British Library

ISBN 1-85315-677-9

Distribution in Europe and Rest of World:

Marston Book Services Ltd
PO Box 269
Abingdon
Oxon OX14 4YN, UK
Tel: +44 (0)1235 465500
Fax: +44 (0)1235 465555
Email: direct.order@marston.co.uk

Distribution in the USA and Canada:

Royal Society of Medicine Press Ltd
c/o BookMasters, Inc,
30 Amberwood Parkway
Ashland, Ohio 44805, USA
Tel: +1 800 247 6553/+1 800 266 5564
Fax: +1 419 281 6883
Email: order@bookmasters.com

Distribution in Australia and New Zealand:

Elsevier Australia
30-52 Smidmore Street
Marrikville NSW 2204, Australia
Tel: +61 2 9349 5811
Fax: +61 2 9349 5911
Email: service@elsevier.com.au

Typeset by Macmillan India Ltd, Bangalore 560025, India

Printed and bound in Great Britain by Bell & Bain Ltd, Glasgow

Introduction to Telemedicine

Second edition

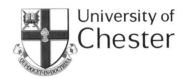

Other titles in telemedicine and e-health from RSM Press

Series Editor
Richard Wootton

Home Telehealth (2006)
Eds: R Wootton, S Dimmick and JC Kvedar, RSM Press, ISBN 1-85315-657-4

Teleneurology (2005)
Eds: R Wootton and V Patterson, RSM Press, ISBN 1-85315-671-X

Telepediatrics: Telemedicine and Child Health (2004)
Eds: R Wootton and J Batch, RSM Press, ISBN 1-85315-645-0

Telepsychiatry and e-Mental Health (2003)
Eds: R Wootton, P Yellowlees and P McLaren, RSM Press, ISBN 1-85315-549-7

Teledermatology (2002)
Eds: R Wootton and AMM Oakley, RSM Press, ISBN 1-85315-507-1

The Legal and Ethical Aspects of Telemedicine (1998)
BA Stanberry, RSM Press, ISBN 1-85315-345-0

Journal of Telemedicine and Telecare
Eds: R Wootton and E Krupinski, RSM Press, ISSN 1357-633X
Publishes peer-reviewed papers on all aspects of telemedicine and telecare.

▶ Contents

Section 4: Other Aspects of Telemedicine 133

▶ List of Contributors

Nancy A Brown, Evidence-based Practice Center, Oregon Health and Science University, Portland, Oregon, USA

John Craig, Department of Neurology, Royal Victoria Hospital, Belfast, UK

Vernon R Curran, Faculty of Medicine, Memorial University of Newfoundland, Canada

Vincenzo Della Mea, Department of Mathematics and Computer Science, University of Udine, Udine, Italy

Gary C Doolittle, Department of Internal Medicine, Division of Hematology/Oncology, Kansas University Medical Center, Kansas City, USA

James Ferguson, Accident and Emergency Department, Aberdeen Royal Infirmary, UK

Brett Harnett, Center for Surgical Innovation, University of Cincinnati, Ohio, USA

Paul J Heinzelmann, Partners Telemedicine, Partners HealthCare System, Boston, and Department of Dermatology, Massachusetts General Hospital, Harvard Medical School, Boston, Massachusetts, USA

N M Hjelm, Department of Chemical Pathology, St George's Hospital, London, UK

Joseph C Kvedar, Partners Telemedicine, Partners HealthCare System, Boston, and Department of Dermatology, Massachusetts General Hospital, Harvard Medical School, Boston, Massachusetts, USA

Nancy E Lugn, Partners Telemedicine, Partners HealthCare System, Boston, Massachusetts, USA

Victor Patterson, Department of Neurology, Royal Victoria Hospital, Belfast, UK; and Centre for Online Health, University of Queensland, Brisbane, Australia

Ryan J Spaulding, Kansas University Medical Center, Kansas City, USA

Benedict Stanberry, Avienda Limited, Cardiff, UK

Paul Taylor, Centre for Health Informatics and Multiprofessional Education, University College London, London, UK

Richard Wootton, Centre for Online Health, University of Queensland, Brisbane, Australia

Peter Yellowlees, Academic Information Systems, University of California Davis, California, USA

▶ Foreword to the First Edition

One of a clinician's truly chastening experiences is finding out that they've missed the diagnosis because they'd never heard about the disease. After all, that's what all that training was about, damn it; to learn how to sort through all of the known possibilities. Likewise, what clinician doesn't want to offer patients the most effective and efficient available treatments and diagnostic techniques? If you don't know the disease, you can't diagnose it. If you don't know the treatment, you can't offer it.

Telemedicine is a medical modality that too few clinicians are even aware of. To many, it is not much more than a confusing hodge-podge of new vocabulary, hardware, software and systems engineering, policy and legal issues.

The clear aim of this book is to bring the promise and problems of telemedicine into the 'top of the mind awareness' of the people who make decisions about medical care. Upon reading it, practitioners will be able to properly place the powerful new technologies and concepts of telemedicine into their strategic, diagnostic and treatment thinking.

The editors have hand picked the world's cream-of-the-crop teleclinicians and practitioners to convey their wisdom and experience. These are not armchair pundits: they are strategic thinkers, all of whom have extensive experience and current involvement in active clinical telemedicine programmes. Their viewpoints reflect the unique and varied experiences of telemedicine programme developers from Australia and Hong Kong to Europe and North America. From them, the reader can learn how to bring rapidly evolving technologies to bear on their own healthcare enterprise, how best to face the challenges of deploying telemedicine, and perhaps most important, how to avoid the pitfalls inherent in moving a massive, lumbering, often hide-bound healthcare system onto a different course.

Telemedicine addresses the key issues that challenge medical practice at the turn of the century: maximizing efficiency while maintaining or improving quality of service, lowering costs, improving access to care, improving access to information, and assuring patient confidentiality and professional accountability. There is no other technique or systems engineering strategy that has the promise of addressing these issues in as global and cost-effective way as telemedicine. Over the past forty years there has been an increasing cascade of pilot projects, public and private programmes (both self-sustaining and externally supported), transnational ventures, and peer-reviewed research studies. For the 'old timer' in the field, the onslaught of information is bewildering. For the newcomer, it may be paralyzing – especially since the technology itself is changing so rapidly that a plan formulated around today's technology may be obsolescent tomorrow.

This book will be of great service to the bewildered and the paralysed. Although technology continues to develop rapidly, the fundamental principles of modern healthcare delivery are slower to change. The contributors to this book do an excellent job of informing the reader about what we know, what we don't know, and what we may expect in the next few years, so that decisions about deploying (often expensive) new technologies are made rationally and with the maximum chance of producing health care which is more efficient and affordable.

The authors are graceful communicators whose accumulated experience offers a guide to bringing into the everyday practice of healthcare the telecommunications technologies that have affected so many other parts of our lives.

Ace Allen
Kansas University Medical Center
1999

▶ Preface to the First Edition

This is an introductory text. Apart from being an introduction for anyone interested in telemedicine, the aim of the book is principally to permit those who are involved in delivering health care, irrespective of their own particular area of interest, to begin to assess how telemedicine might be applied to their working practice. In particular it is addressed to those who have actual contact with consumers, i.e. patients and others. Considering how busy most health care workers are, it is unlikely that many of them will wish to become instant 'experts' in information and telecommunications technology, and we have therefore omitted large quantities of technical detail. Likewise an introductory text, whose aim is to present telemedicine in all its diversity to as wide an audience of health care workers as possible, is hardly the place to discuss such areas as future policies or standards for telemedicine. To give too much space to these issues, however important in due course, is more likely to discourage the average doctor, nurse, or other health care worker from considering telemedicine as a means of improving care in their area of interest. These topics are therefore only touched on very briefly.

In order to make the book as practically relevant as possible, contributors have been selected who have extensive practical experience of telemedicine and, in some cases, have also set up sustainable telemedicine programmes. The book is divided into four sections:

1. An introductory section giving an overview of telemedicine in its broadest sense and outlining the requirements for a telemedicine system to deliver health care by this method.
2. A section describing the areas where telemedicine is currently being used to assist health care.
3. A section on how to assess whether or not telemedicine might have anything to offer to a particular field of health care delivery, how to go about developing such a telemedicine service and how to determine its effects. In keeping with the practical approach, a chapter is also included about how to perform a real-time interactive videoconsultation.
4. A concluding section summarizing the benefits of telemedicine, but also highlighting potential problems. With regard to the latter, a chapter on the relevant medicolegal issues in telemedicine and how these might be addressed is included. Finally, before a look to the future of telemedicine is attempted, a chapter is included on sources of information for this exciting new means of health care delivery.

We hope you enjoy reading it.

Belfast, 1999   Richard Wootton
John Craig

▶ Preface to the Second Edition

The first edition of *Introduction to Telemedicine* remained in print for about five years and found favour as a student text. A second edition has therefore been prepared. All the chapters have been revised and updated, and more recent references have been cited where appropriate. Not all of the original authors could be contacted, so some new authors have kindly agreed to contribute. However, the structure of the first edition has been retained.

Since the first edition of this book, the Royal Society of Medicine Press has published a number of titles on different aspects of telemedicine. This introductory text therefore forms the first in a series of readings, suitable for students and others interested in an overview of telemedicine. Although the terms used to describe telemedicine have expanded since the first edition, we believe that the principles remain the same. Whether the activity is described as telemedicine, telehealth, online health or e-health is immaterial; what matters is that people undertaking those activities should understand the basis for successful telemedical practice.

April 2006

Richard Wootton
Brisbane
John Craig, Victor Patterson
Belfast

Section 1: Background

1. **Introduction to the practice of telemedicine**
   John Craig and Victor Patterson

2. **Telemedicine systems and telecommunications**
   Brett Hamett

▶1

Introduction to the practice of telemedicine

John Craig and Victor Patterson

Introduction

One of the great challenges facing humankind in the 21st century is to make high-quality health care available to all. Such a vision has been expressed by the World Health Organization (WHO) in its health-for-all strategy in the 21st century.[1] Realizing this vision will be difficult, perhaps impossible, because of the burdens imposed on a growing world population by old and new diseases, rising expectations for health, and socioeconomic conditions that have, if anything, increased disparities in health status between and within countries.

Traditionally, part of the difficulty in achieving equitable access to health care has been that the provider and the recipient must be present in the same place and at the same time. Recent advances in information and communication technologies, however, have created unprecedented opportunities for overcoming this by increasing the number of ways that health care can be delivered. This applies both to developing countries with weak or unstable economies and to industrialized countries. The possibilities for using information and communication technologies to improve health-care delivery ('health telematics') are increasingly being recognized. The WHO has stated that with regard to its health-for-all strategy it recommends that the WHO and its member states should:

> ...integrate the appropriate use of health telematics in the overall policy and strategy for the attainment of health for all in the 21st century, thus fulfilling the vision of a world in which the benefits of science, technology and public health development are made equitably available to all people everywhere.[2]

Such a commitment to improve health-care delivery, by utilizing information and telecommunications technologies, is also being considered by those with the financial means to do so, for example, the participants in various European Commission projects. At the national and subnational level, there is also evidence of governmental interest in the benefits that these technologies might bring to health care. For example, in the UK, information technology including telemedicine is at the heart of the government's strategy to modernize and improve the NHS.[3] Telemedicine, the area where medicine and information and telecommunications technology meet, is probably the part of this revolution that could have the greatest impact on health-care delivery.

What is telemedicine?

Telemedicine is the delivery of health care and the exchange of health-care information across distances. The prefix 'tele' derives from the Greek for 'at a distance'; hence, more simply, telemedicine is medicine at a distance. As such, it encompasses the whole range of medical activities including diagnosis, treatment and prevention of disease, continuing education of health-care providers and consumers, and research and evaluation.

Telecare is a related term and refers to the provision, at a distance, of nursing and community support to a patient. Similarly, telehealth refers to public health services delivered at a distance, to people who are not necessarily unwell, but who wish to remain well and independent. In effect, however, despite repeated discussions about what constitutes telemedicine, telecare and telehealth and what their differences are, all involve the transfer of information about health-related issues between one or more sites, so that the health of individuals and their communities can be advanced. In other words, the information is moved, not the providers or the recipients of health care. Nowadays, the transfer of information is generally facilitated by the use of some kind of telecommunications network. An umbrella term encompassing all health-related activities carried out over a distance by such information and communication technologies is 'health telematics'. With this in mind, telemedicine, as an integral part of health telematics, might be defined as:

> Rapid access to shared and remote medical expertise by means of telecommunications and information technologies, no matter where the patient or the relevant information is located.[4]

What telemedicine is not

Telemedicine is not a technology or a separate or new branch of medicine, or for that matter even new. It is also not the panacea that will cure all of the world's health-related problems or a means by which health-care workers can be replaced. It is also not an activity for antiquarians or Luddites, who range from those who are simply not at ease with the use of electronic machinery, right through to those who feel that telemedicine threatens the very fabric of the practice of medicine, and as such should be actively opposed. Equally, however, it is not the sole territory of 'computer nerds' or 'technophiles'. In fact, the tendency of these individuals to concentrate on the technical rather than the practical when discussing telemedicine may explain the antipathy of some clinicians towards practising medicine this way. Sensible, practical presentations by those who have actual experience of telemedicine have the potential to change the minds of those health-care workers who feel that telemedicine is not for them, either because it is 'gimmicky', industry-driven and therefore 'less than respectable', or unfathomable. Finally, and probably most important, for the most part telemedicine is far from being a mature discipline, and much work remains to be done to establish its place in health-care delivery.

Types of telemedicine

The common thread for all telemedicine applications is that a client of some kind (e.g. patient or health-care worker) obtains an opinion from someone with more expertise in the relevant field, when the parties are separated in space, in time or both. Telemedicine episodes may be classified on the basis of:

- the interaction between the client and the expert and
- the type of information being transmitted.

The *type of interaction* is usually classified as either prerecorded (also called store-and-forward) or realtime (also called synchronous). In the former, information is acquired and stored in some format, before being sent, by an appropriate means, for expert interpretation at some later time. Email is a common method of store-and-forward interaction. In contrast, in realtime interactions, there is no appreciable delay between the information being collected, transmitted and displayed. Interactive communication between individuals at the sites is therefore possible. Videoconferencing is a common method of realtime interaction.

The *information transmitted* between the two sites can take many forms, including data and text, audio, still images and video pictures. Combining the type of interaction and the type of information to be transmitted allows telemedicine episodes to be classified as in Figure 1.1. In certain applications, such as teleradiology, a technique that involves the transmission of digital radiographs between institutions, it is possible for the interaction to be either prerecorded or realtime; the latter requires that the expert be available to give an opinion as the image is taken and transmitted. Prerecorded and realtime telemedicine applications are discussed in Chapters 3 and 4.

		Information transmitted	
		Still images	Moving images (video)
Interaction	Realtime		e.g. telepsychiatry
	Prerecorded	e.g. teleradiology	

Figure 1.1 Classification system for telemedicine episodes

History of telemedicine

Most telemedicine has clearly occurred in the last 20–30 years, concomitant with advances in information technology. If, however, telemedicine is considered to be any medical activity performed at a distance, irrespective of how the information is transmitted, its history is much older. An early example of medicine at a distance, perhaps one of the first public health surveillance networks, was in the Middle Ages, when information about bubonic plague was transmitted across Europe by such means as bonfires. With developments in national postal services in the mid-19th century, the means by which more personal health-care delivery at a distance could be performed was facilitated, and the practice of physicians providing diagnosis, and directions for a cure, was established.

In the mid-19th century, telegraphy – signalling by wires – also began and was quickly deployed by those providing and planning for medical care. This included its use in the American Civil War to transmit casualty lists and order medical supplies, with later technological developments permitting X-ray images to be transmitted. In much of Europe and the USA, the telegraph was rapidly superseded by the telephone as a general means of communication, but in Australia it survived for much longer because of the enormous distances involved.

The telephone has been used for delivering health services since its invention in the late 19th century, and for 50 or so years remained the mainstay of communication for such purposes. However, it was realized as early as 1910 that the telephone could be used for purposes other than voice communication; amplified sounds from a stethoscope were transmitted through the telephone network and similar devices are still used today. Other uses for the ordinary telephone network have since been realized and include the transmission of electrocardiograms (ECGs) and electroencephalograms (EEGs).

The next development of widespread significance was at the end of the 19th century when communication by radio became possible. This was done initially by Morse code and later by voice. Use of the radio to provide medical advice for seafarers was recognized very quickly, and in 1920 the Seaman's Church Institute of New York became one of the first organizations to provide medical care using the radio, with at least another five maritime nations establishing radio medical services by 1938. One of these was the International Radio Medical Centre (CIRM), whose headquarters are in Rome, Italy. It was set up in 1935 and in its first 60 years assisted with over 42,000 patients, making it the largest single organization in the world to use telemedicine to provide health care to seafarers.[5] Radio medical advice for passengers on long-distance air journeys has also been provided more recently. For in-flight medical incidents that require professional assistance, and which occur at a rate of about 1 in 50,000 passengers carried, assistance can be obtained from on-call health-care workers on the ground.

The birth of modern telemedicine

The recent development of telemedicine has been facilitated on two fronts. First, there are the advances in electronic methods of communication. Initially, analogue methods were used, but now modern digital communication techniques are the mainstay. Second, telemedicine has developed because of the pioneering efforts of a few organizations and individuals. The former generally represented the interest of high-tech ventures, such as the manned space-flight programme of the National Aeronautics and Space Administration (NASA) in the USA. While these were no doubt of great importance in fostering the development of telemedicine and telecommunications generally, the efforts of a few individuals using readily-available commercial equipment have arguably been just as important for the development of telemedicine. It is interesting to note that in the 40 or so years since these individuals initiated their ventures things have changed relatively little, as far as who is doing research of practical value, and how it is being done.

A major influence on the development of telemedicine was the introduction of television. By the late 1950s, developments in closed-circuit television and video communications were made use of by medical personnel, who began to employ them in clinical situations. As early as 1964, a two-way closed-circuit television system was set up between the Nebraska Psychiatric Institute in Omaha and the state mental hospital in Norfolk, 112 miles (180 km) away.[6] The system permitted interactive consultations between specialists and general practitioners, and facilitated education and training at the distant site. Another early example of television linking doctors and patients was at the Massachusetts General Hospital/Logan International Airport Medical Station, which was established in 1967.[7] This used a two-way audiovisual microwave circuit and permitted care to be provided to passengers and airport employees 24 h a day by nurses, supplemented by physician expertise using the audiovisual link. In an early report of the feasibility of this method of delivering health care, the observations of 1000 episodes were documented. It is noteworthy that few reports of telemedicine projects since have contained such numbers of episodes performed. More recently, there has been a major growth in realtime telemedicine with the wide availability of videoconferencing. This has been made possible because of improvements in digital communications and the introduction of low-cost computing, many of the videoconferencing systems now being based on PCs (see Chapter 2).

The recent developments of mobile phones and satellite communications have allowed mobile telemedicine. Early examples of such programmes were the Alaska ATS-6 Satellite Biomedical Demonstration from 1971 to 1975, which assessed the viability of improving village health care in Alaska using satellite-mediated video consultation,[8] and the Memorial University of Newfoundland programme established in 1977, initially to provide distance education as well as medical care to Canadians.[9]

Where is telemedicine being done?

Today, telemedicine represents the experiences, opinions, perceptions and interests of a vast number of individuals and organizations. Most operational telemedicine services, of which the majority concern diagnosis and clinical management at a distance, are in industrialized countries, especially the USA, Canada, Australia and the UK. Telemedicine also includes tele-education, which is discussed further in Chapter 5, and distance treatment, e.g. telesurgery. The latter area remains the subject of media interest, but there is little practical experience. Teleradiology is the branch of telemedicine which has been integrated best into the fabric of clinical practice. So well integrated is it that figures on its use are impossible to come by.

A recent survey of teleconsultation activity (excluding teleradiology) in the USA found that over 85,000 teleconsultations were done in 2002, performed by more than 200 programmes, in over 30 specialties.[10] Mental health, paediatrics, dermatology, cardiology and orthopaedics accounted for almost 60% of these teleconsultations, with approximately 50% using interactive video, the rest prerecorded or non-video technology (Figure 1.2).

This survey also identified 52 telemedicine programmmes outside the USA, with Canada (10), Australia (9) and the UK (9) being the major contributors. Elsewhere in Europe, Norway has a National Centre for Telemedicine based at Tromsø and both Finland and Russia have functioning telemedicine programmes. Hong Kong has established programmes in the rehabilitation of older people,[11] and there is a telemedicine service for burns patients in Australia.[12] In South America, Argentina has seen its telemedicine applications collapse.[13]

Despite most telemedical services being concentrated in industrialized countries, there are several lines of evidence to suggest their adoption globally, including within developing countries. The first of these is witnessed in the number of conferences and meetings that are occurring with increasing frequency throughout the world, and the diversity of nations that are represented at them. Africa epitomizes the paradox of telemedicine, that the areas that would benefit most from it do not have the resources to utilize it. There are functioning networks in South Africa and in Mali,[14] the latter linked to a hospital in Geneva. There are several other telemedicine networks linking the industrialized and developing worlds; including those run by the Swinfen Charitable Trust[15] and the Medical Missions for Children.[16] This is an area that is likely to grow in the future.

Research

The output of papers on telemedicine-related subjects as indexed on MEDLINE has been fairly constant at about 1000 papers annually over the last five

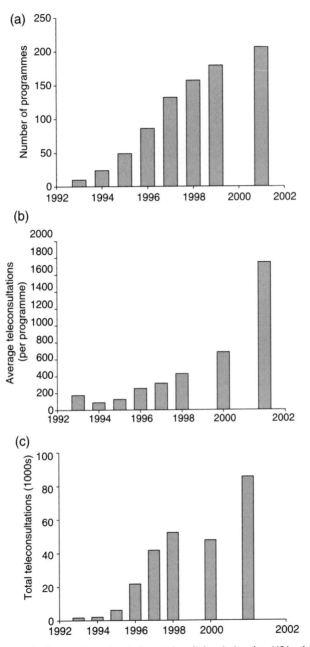

Figure 1.2 Teleconsultation activity (excluding teleradiology) in the USA. (a) Number of telemedicine programmes; (b) average number of teleconsultations per programme; (c) total number of teleconsultations in the USA each year. Data from Grigsby[10]

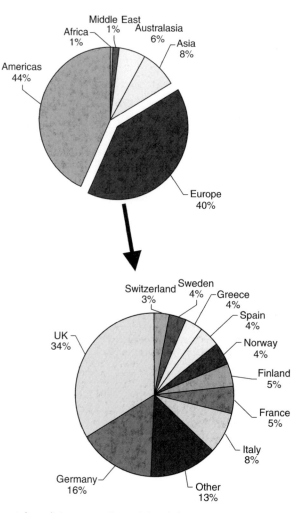

Figure 1.3 Primary telemedicine research – origin of the research papers published in the two specialist telemedicine journals (*Telemedicine Journal and e-Health* and *Journal of Telemedicine and Telecare*) from 1998–2003 (*n* = 2952)

years.[17,18] Prior to that, there had been a period of rapid growth in annual output from about 100 in 1994. Although almost 50% of recent papers originate in the USA, Finland and Norway produce the greatest number of publications per head of population (Figure 1.3). One specialist journal, *Journal of Telemedicine and Telecare*, published 13% of all papers but, encouragingly, over 50% of MEDLINE-indexed journals have published at least one article on telemedicine.[17] There has been an increasing number of randomized controlled trials published[19,20] and also some systematic reviews. The results of the latter are rather critical of much of the telemedicine literature, and one even suggests that much of it should not have passed the peer-review process.[21] The correspondence subsequent to this review did question the relevance of such academically rigorous analyses to telemedicine, the aim of which is not to replace face-to-face medicine and take over the world, but more usually to improve people's health in certain well defined situations. Telemedicine has a number of separate attributes – feasibility, acceptability, cost, effectiveness, safety, sustainability – and the importance of studying each of these systematically will vary from application to application. For example, to use telemedicine to support an Antarctic expedition requires only that feasibility be demonstrated, since acceptability and cost are less relevant. In contrast, using telemedicine for a single specialty in a large region needs considerably more attributes to be studied. The paradox here is that if research is tightly controlled to meet the strict requirements of the writers of systematic reviews, it may become less relevant to real-life situations and therefore less likely to be introduced into clinical practice.

Why is telemedicine being done?

The frequent references to telemedicine in the medical and lay literature and the increasing number of politicians who appear to be interested in its use are very noticeable. McLaren and Ball have argued that the reason for such interest is that 'Technology has the power to mesmerise. It is for this reason that telemedicine has a high profile'.[22] While there is no doubt that for some this is true, there are basically two reasons why telemedicine should be used:

- there is no alternative to telemedicine;
- telemedicine is better than existing conventional services.

No alternative to telemedicine
Telemedicine clearly has a role in the case of emergencies in remote environments such as the Antarctic and in ships or aeroplanes, where it may be difficult, if not impossible, to get medical care to the patient in time. In countries with unstable or weak economies, however, where health-care services are often not a priority, telemedicine also permits access to services that would not otherwise be available. An example is the provision of medical services from the city of Arkhangelsk in northwest Russia to other parts of the region and exchange of knowledge and experience between the University Hospital of Tromsø, in northern Norway, and northwest Russia.[23]

Telemedicine is better
Telemedicine has obvious advantages in remote or rural areas where it improves access to health services, obviating the need for patients and health-care workers to travel. Even in urban areas, however, telemedicine can improve access to health services and to information. Telemedicine has also been shown to improve

the consistency and quality of health care.[24] It may sometimes also be cheaper than conventional practice, although, as previously mentioned, scientifically sound economic appraisals of telemedicine applications are only just beginning to appear.

Other reasons why telemedicine is being done

Telemedicine is occasionally accused of being an 'industry' driven by commercial rather than consumer interests. Certainly, of the numerous experimental and operational telemedicine systems in use, or at the drawing-board stage, some would appear to have been set up primarily to produce financial benefits for the providers (individuals or organizations) of the service, rather than health benefits for the consumers. Telemedicine principally practised for financial gain is not confined to the manufacturers of equipment, but includes health-care workers (real or fraudulent), telecommunications networks and other organizations. The technological advances that have been necessary to develop telemedicine to its current state, or which are likely to occur in the future, are driven mainly by market forces; hence, there is a concern that the reputation of telemedicine as a whole could be damaged by the actions of those aiming to make their fortune. This is especially likely if operational services are set up without prior establishment of the need for a particular application in a certain setting, and evidence that the service as established is effective and cost-effective. If there was ever an argument for the need for research for all telemedicine applications prior to widespread adoption, this is surely it.

Effects of telemedicine

In broad terms, telemedicine can be expected to improve equity of access to health care, the quality of that care and the efficiency by which it is delivered, by enhancing communication up and down the health-care pyramid. Widespread adoption of telemedicine would permit decentralization; work previously done in the secondary sector, for example, could be performed in primary care and work previously done in the primary care sector could be devolved to the community level (Figure 1.4). Such changes, if implemented in the developing world, could potentially have the greatest effect, allowing under-served people to benefit from a greatly improved standard of health care. In all remote or rural areas, however, telemedicine could have a great impact, permitting among other opportunities, better diagnostic and therapeutic services, faster and easier access to medical knowledge, and enhanced communication between health-care workers.

Conclusion

There is no doubt that telemedicine is effective in certain situations. The transition to a world where telemedicine is employed to the maximum will not be

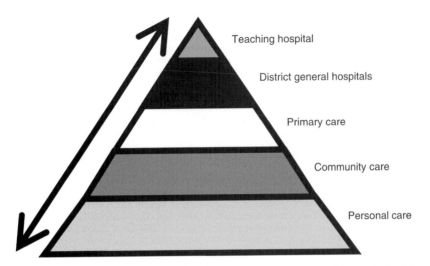

Figure 1.4 Telemedicine as a means for improving communication up and down the health-care pyramid

realized, however, if governments and health-care organizations do not produce strategies to encourage its development. Wootton has summarized the critical issues that will need to be addressed in such strategies as part of a fourfold commitment: to encourage and provide funding for telemedicine research; to develop a plan for implementation (once clinical effectiveness and cost-effectiveness have been demonstrated); to assess the major structural changes required within organizations to incorporate this method of delivering health care; to develop a process for training, formulation of practice guidelines, quality control and continuing audit.[25] Other issues that will need to be addressed include ethical and medicolegal concerns, human and cultural factors, such as resistance to change, lack of infrastructure, linguistic differences and illiteracy, and technical and organizational factors. None of these should be insurmountable.

References

1   World Health Organization. *Health-for-all Policy for the 21st Century, HQ* (document EB101/8). Geneva: WHO, 1997
2   World Health Organization. *A Health Telematics Policy* (document DGO/98.1). Geneva: WHO, 1998
3   NHS Executive. *Information for Health: An Information Strategy for the Modern NHS*. London: The Stationery Office, 1998
4   CEC DG XIII. *Research and Technology Development on Telematics Systems in Health Care AIM 1993*. Annual Technical Report on RTD: Health Care. Brussels, 1993
5   Amenta F, Rizzo N. Maritime radiomedical services. In: Wootton R, ed. *European Telemedicine 1998/99*. London: Kensington Publications, 1999:125–6

6 Benschoter RA, Wittson CL, Ingham CG. Teaching and consultation by television: I. Closed-circuit collaboration. *J Hosp Commun Psychiatry* 1965;**16**:99–100

7 Murphy RLH, Bird KT. Telediagnosis: a new community health resource. Observations on the feasibility of telediagnosis based on 1000 patient transactions. *Am J Public Health* 1974;**64**:113–19

8 Foote DR. Satellite communication for rural health care in Alaska. *J Commun* 1977;**27**:173–82

9 Elford R. Telemedicine activities at Memorial University of Newfoundland: a historical review, 1975–1997. *Telemed J* 1998;**6**:207–24

10 Grigsby B. *2004 TRC Report on US Telemedicine Activity*. Kingston, NJ: Civic Research Institute, 2004

11 Lai JC, Woo J, Hui E, Chan WM. Telerehabilitation – a new model for community-based stroke rehabilitation. *J Telemed Telecare* 2004;**10**:199–205

12 Smith AC, Youngberry K, Mill J, Kimble R, Wootton R. A review of three years experience using email and videoconferencing for the delivery of post-acute burns care to children in Queensland. *Burns* 2004;**30**:248–52

13 Urtubey X, Petrich M. Argentina's national telemedicine programme: reasons for a premature failure. *J Telemed Telecare* 2002;**8** (Suppl. 3):69–71

14 Geissbuhler A, Ly O, Lovis C, L'Haire JF. Telemedicine in Western Africa: lessons learned from a pilot project in Mali, perspectives and recommendations. *AMIA Annu Symp Proc* 2003:249–53

15 Vassallo DJ, Hoque F, Farquarson Roberts M, Patterson V, Swinfen P, Swinfen R. An evaluation of the first year's experience with a low-cost telemedicine link in Bangladesh. *J Telemed Telecare* 2001;**7**:125–38

16 Reznik M, Marcin JP, Ozuah P. Telemedicine and underserved communities in developing nations. In: Wootton R, Batch J, eds. *Telepediatrics*. London: RSM Press, 2004:193–98

17 Moser PL, Hauffe H, Lorenz IH, *et al*. Publication output in telemedicine during the period January 1964 to July 2003. *J Telemed Telecare* 2004;**10**:72–7

18 Youngberry K. Telemedicine research and MEDLINE. *J Telemed Telecare* 2004;**10**:121–3

19 Wootton R, Bloomer SE, Corbett R, *et al*. Multicentre randomised control trial comparing real time teledermatology with conventional outpatient dermatological care: societal cost-benefit analysis. *Br Med J* 2000;**320**:1252–6

20 Chua R, Craig J, Wootton R, Patterson V. Randomised controlled trial of telemedicine for new neurological outpatient referrals. *J Neurol Neurosurg Psychiatry* 2001;**71**:63–6

21 Whitten PS, Mair FS, Haycox A, May CR, Williams TL, Hellmich S. Systematic review of cost effectiveness studies of telemedicine interventions. *Br Med J* 2002;**324**:1434–7

22 McLaren P, Ball CJ. Telemedicine: lessons remain unheeded. *Br Med J* 1995;**310**:1390–1

23 Sørensen T, Rundhovde A, Kozlov VD. Telemedicine in north-west Russia. *J Telemed Telecare* 1999;**5**:153–6

24 Darkins A, Dearden CH, Rocke LG, Martin JB, Sibson L, Wootton R. An evaluation of telemedical support for a minor treatment centre. *J Telemed Telecare* 1996;**2**:93–9

25 Wootton R. Telemedicine in the National Health Service. *J Roy Soc Med* 1998;**91**:614–21

▶2

Telemedicine systems and telecommunications

Brett Harnett

Introduction

The practice of telemedicine can be divided into two distinct categories: realtime and store-and-forward. Realtime telemedicine involves synchronous inter-action between the parties concerned. For example, a health-care professional and a patient may interact by videoconferencing. While realtime telemedicine is often effective in terms of consultation and patient satisfaction,[1,2] it presents challenges. Foremost is the scheduling of the parties concerned, because there are usually two health-care providers involved in the consultation (the local provider and the remote physician), and they both need to be available at the same time.

In contrast, store-and-forward (S&F) telemedicine is an asynchronous interaction, so that a clinical query, for example, can be transmitted by the referrer and then answered by a specialist at a convenient time. Email is a common example of this type of telemedicine. Although diagnostic accuracy may be lower with S&F telemedicine, it is advantageous from the point of view of cost, complexity and convenience.[3]

The field of telemedicine encompasses more than clinical interactions, of course. Having the technology to connect remote sites also allows distance learning. This may involve training or information sharing for health-care professionals that does not directly involve patients but still enhances care.

Essential components of a telemedicine system

Successful telemedicine requires appropriate equipment and some kind of telecommunications medium. However, successful telemedicine requires more than just technology. The three essential components are:

(1) the personnel,
(2) the technology,
(3) a liberal measure of perseverance.

Personnel

For any telemedicine system to work in practice – in a real clinical situation – suitable, committed personnel are essential. People with the necessary skills to undertake the clinical components are required at both ends of any telemedicine link. This means that there must be trained staff at the referring end of the link who are able to handle the patient contact required. They must be comfortable with this mode of care delivery and they will probably need prior training, since telemedicine will represent a clinical situation that they are not normally exposed to (see Chapter 6 for further discussion of this point). Unless this is planned in advance, the technology may be under-used (or even ignored entirely) by staff who may be uncomfortable with the new processes.

At the specialist, or consulting, end of a telemedicine link, different characteristics are required of the personnel. The two most important factors are the reliability of the equipment and the availability of the appropriate personnel. Use of a telemedicine system will decrease if the patient information is available but the link is unusable, either for technical reasons or because the appropriate staff are not available at the diagnostic end. It is essential to ensure that there are sufficient trained personnel and that the schedules are carefully planned to enable links to be used with minimum delays, even in emergencies. Training is a very important factor in successful telemedicine.[4]

Technology

The technology is in many ways the most straightforward part of a telemedicine system and, once a working link has been established, it can largely be ignored. Much of the equipment required may already be available for other purposes, and can be shared if planned properly. Reliability is a requirement for all medical equipment and telemedicine equipment is no exception. For telemedicine, all the equipment needs to function properly, since any malfunction will break the chain required for a successful link. Although modern computers and operating systems are fairly reliable, the integration of components still requires close attention to ensure reliability and ease of use. Unreliable technology is likely to cause the system to be under-used or even ignored.

Perseverance

Finally, it is important to mention one crucial component, without which a telemedicine system will not function. Experience shows that at least one dedicated and committed individual is needed with the perseverance to overcome the inertia inherent in all established clinical routines, and the commitment to champion the new system until it can demonstrate its usefulness (see Chapters 6 and 7). This mentor or champion of the system will help to drive the implementation and to deal with problems as they arise.[5]

Clinical requirements

The technology required for a telemedicine link can be divided into three categories:

(1) equipment to capture the clinical information at each site,
(2) the telecommunications link needed to transmit this information between the sites,
(3) equipment to display the information at each site.

Before the technology can be selected, it is necessary to consider the nature of the information to be transmitted between the sites, because this will determine the choice of equipment and the telecommunications network. Factors to be considered include:

(1) the types of information to be transmitted,
(2) the quantity of information to be transferred,
(3) security and privacy (e.g. in Europe and the USA there has been recent legislation about data security).

Types of information to be transmitted

Different clinical situations generate very different types of clinical information (Table 2.1). Hence, there are many possible sources of data that can be used in telemedicine applications. In some cases this can be relatively simple information, such as concentrations of a metabolite (e.g. a high blood glucose concentration may suggest diabetes), whereas in others more qualitative and subtle information is needed, as in psychiatric assessments, where observations of posture, speech and mental state are required. Not all information will be needed at every site. For example, a telepsychiatry application will probably require ordinary commercial videoconferencing equipment instead of very high-quality audio or video signals and a telemonitoring service will require only data and text transfer, without audio and video.

The clinical need for any telemedicine project must be carefully assessed before making decisions about what equipment will be required. In the past, projects have been established on the assumption that it will be necessary to transmit all possible types of information. This can lead to disproportionately high set-up and maintenance costs that may not be justified by the actual telemedicine use. In general, it is preferable to limit the initial system to a defined clinical goal and so minimize the costs.

Quantity of information transferred

The units in which the quantity of digital information is measured are the bit and the Byte (Box 2.1). One method by which the total volume of information can be reduced is to compress it first, and then decompress it on reception. This is not always an acceptable technique for medicolegal reasons (i.e. only the original raw signal may be considered acceptable).

Table 2.1 Examples of clinical information

Information source	Type	Typical file size
Electronic stethoscope	Audio	100 kByte
ECG recording	Data	100 kByte
Chest X-ray	Still image	1 MByte
Fetal ultrasound recording (30 s)	Moving images (video)	10 MByte

---

Box 2.1 Bits and Bytes

A Byte of digital information corresponds approximately to a single character of alphabetical text. So, for example, a page of text comprising 50 lines, each of 60 characters (and spaces), contains 3000 characters altogether. It can therefore be represented in a computer by approximately 3000 Bytes of information, i.e. about 3 kByte. A floppy disk commonly stores 1.4 MByte (i.e. 1400 kByte) of information and PC hard disks often have capacities of 10–40 GByte (i.e. 10,000–40,000 MByte).

Each Byte is normally represented in the computer by eight binary digits or bits (0 or 1 signals). Thus, to transmit 3000 Bytes of information, a total of 24,000 bits of data would have to be sent. Telecommunications line speeds are usually quoted in bit/s. For example, a modem connected to the telephone network can normally transmit information at speeds of 28–56,000 bits per second. The 3000 Bytes representing a page of text would therefore take something like 1 s to send (the *actual* speed of information transmission is always much lower than the *theoretical* speed, because of the necessity for transmission line protocols).

Authors should distinguish carefully between bits and Bytes, which represent a frequent source of confusion in telemedicine.

A careful assessment of the above needs will determine the quantity of information that must be transmitted between the project sites, and the time frame over which it must be sent to achieve the desired clinical goals. In S&F applications, the transmission time may not be important; in realtime applications, the transmission time is usually critical.

Once this fundamental aspect has been established, it will then be possible to assess whether there is a technically feasible means of achieving it. In practice, some solution is almost always possible, but the costs may not be justified by the clinical benefit.

Information capture

The types of information that are relevant to telemedicine can be divided into five broad categories:

- documents,
- electronic medical records,
- still images,
- audio,
- video.

Documents

Documentary information (e.g. reports, letters or static medical records) can be transmitted in digital form if the information already exists as a computer text file. Alternatively, paper documents can be digitized using a flatbed scanner or a document camera, and then transmitted as still images (see below). Note, however, that, for non-urgent cases, copies of written records can be posted to the consultant end of the link in advance, or paper documents can be faxed before or during a telemedicine session. Even in the age of digital telemedicine, the use of the postal service can represent a very cost-effective way of transferring large quantities of information from one place to another; the disadvantage involves only the delay and the human interaction required.

Electronic medical records

Traditional paper-based records are gradually being replaced by electronic medical records (EMRs). At present, the EMR is a hodge-podge of heterogeneous, proprietary systems that rarely interoperate successfully. Efforts are underway to create a highly interoperable EMR system, where data can flow across the health-care continuum seamlessly.[6,7] EMRs will allow instant access to a patient's record, including the business operations such as billing and reimbursement.

Still images

Two major classes of image are important in telemedicine – those of unspecified quality and those where the diagnostic needs (and hence legal consequences) dictate a particular image quality (Figure 2.1). The difference can best be appreciated by considering the difference between photocopies of images and the originals – a photocopy may be perfectly legible and acceptable for many purposes, but fine detail present in the original may have been lost. For some types of image this can be crucial, and the requirements have been particularly well studied for radiographs.[8]

For many telemedicine purposes, a simple photographic image may be sufficient. For instance, low-cost digital cameras now provide very good imaging quality and may be adequate to capture an image of a skin lesion for teledermatology or a view down a microscope for telepathology.[9] Alternatively, an inexpensive flatbed scanner can be used to digitize photographs or charts such as electrocardiogram (ECG) traces (Figure 2.2). If the scanner is equipped with the appropriate transparency attachment, then 35 mm slides or X-ray films can also be scanned. Where relatively simple diagnoses are required, such basic equipment may be more than adequate, e.g. for emergency room assessment of X-rays of a simple fracture.

Another inexpensive method is to capture still images using a video camera, possibly one that is specially designed for imaging documents (Figure 2.3). In addition, many diagnostic instruments now provide a video output, for example ultrasound scanners. Still images can be recorded with a video capture card on a personal computer (PC) and a suitable screen capture program.

When high-quality diagnostic images are required, the equipment involved can be costly. Modern diagnostic imaging devices are often equipped with digital outputs, which allow images to be transmitted between sites. However, it is common for telemedicine links to be set up in situations where the patient side of the link has old or outdated equipment. In this case, it may be necessary to purchase specialized equipment, such as high-resolution X-ray film digitizers, which are much more expensive (10–20 times) than flatbed scanners designed to work with PCs.

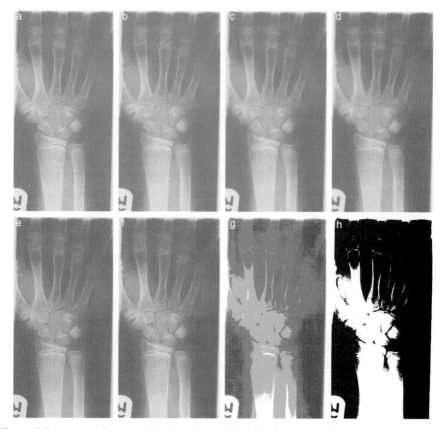

Figure 2.1 Image quality in a still picture is usually defined in terms of the numbers of picture elements in the image (pixels) and the numbers of their black and white – or colour – levels. (a–d) show the same X-ray image digitized at different resolutions: 240, 120, 60, 30 dots/inch. (e–h) show the same X-ray images displayed with different numbers of grey levels per pixel: 255, 15, 5 and 2

Digital Imaging and Communications in Medicine (DICOM) is an established standard for digital image transmission in radiology; it defines how images of clinical quality are distributed via networks.

Audio

At its simplest, voice transmitted by telephone or radio can be used for some remote diagnoses. Although the telephone system has been designed for voice transmission, it is not necessarily ideal for all types of medical sound transmission. Telephones use analogue (Box 2.2) transmission, which is therefore susceptible to noise and loss of quality, especially over long distances. Digital signal transmission offers many advantages, particularly since digital signals can be transmitted over networks for long distances without degradation. It is also possible to process a digital signal in various ways,

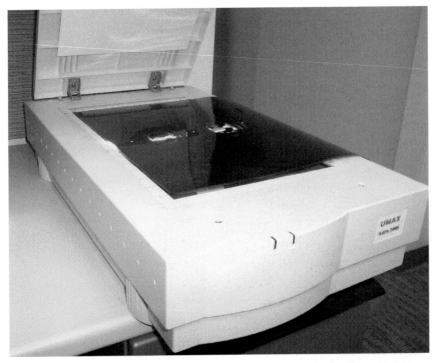

Figure 2.2 A flatbed scanner can be used to digitize a paper record. With a suitable backlight, X-ray films can also be digitized (photo credit: B Harnett)

including compressing it so that a live or recorded voice requires less data to be transmitted than the original signal (see below for further information about compression).

Most modern PCs are equipped with a sound card that is suitable for capturing audio for telemedicine purposes. No special equipment is required other than a suitable microphone. In some cases, it is also possible to connect these cards directly to the equipment that is being used; for example, the audio output of an ultrasound scanner can be connected to the PC. Another option is simply to use an ordinary telephone line as the audio portion of the session. This frees up more bandwidth for video.

Video

A common view of telemedicine is that it only involves realtime video images transmitted between remote sites for the purposes of consultation between a doctor and a patient. This is certainly one form of telemedicine, although it is by no means the only one. In cases where video transmission is considered appropriate, the issue arises of what video quality is required, since unsurprisingly the higher the quality, the higher the cost of the equipment and the transmission. In the majority of applications, commercial videoconferencing units provide the most straightforward solution to the problem of transmitting

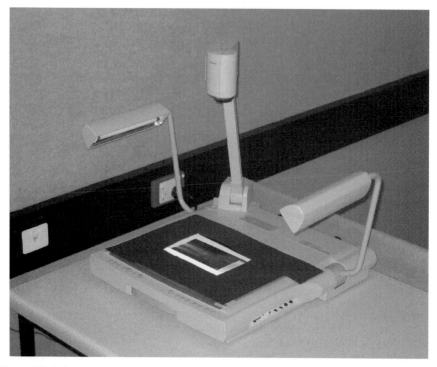

Figure 2.3 A document camera is an alternative method of digitizing X-ray films. Note the use of black cardboard masks around the region of interest

video pictures for telemedicine. Generally speaking, such units provide video pictures that are not as good as broadcast quality television (TV), although in many clinical applications this does not seem to matter.[10] When considering this question, it is worth bearing in mind that the users' opinions will be influenced, even if subconsciously, by the domestic TV that they are used to watching (Box 2.3).

A wide range of telemedicine equipment and accessories is available commercially. A benefit of using commercial suppliers is the technical assistance that they can provide, which includes setting up the working connection and (in most cases) a help desk for technical problems. Many suppliers can perform software upgrades and fault-finding by logging on to the equipment from their home base. For those without technical knowledge or access to in-house technical support, this may be important to the success of a telemedicine project.

Compression of video signals

Commercial videoconferencing units all use compression techniques to reduce the quantity of data being transmitted, and therefore the communication costs. This means that the units at either end of a link must be compatible, i.e. the same compression and decompression algorithms must be employed. To ensure that

---

Box 2.2 Analogue and digital

An *analogue* signal is one whose magnitude is continuously variable. For example, an electrical signal might have a magnitude of about 1.2 V (measured with an inexpensive voltmeter), while a more expensive instrument might show it to be 1.2345 V. The value measured depends on the resolution of the instrument.

In contrast, a *digital* signal can vary – or be measured – only in discrete steps. The digital representation of the same voltage might show it to be 1.2 V the adjacent levels being perhaps 1.0 V and 1.4 V. Increasing the sensitivity of the measurement does not alter the value.

To transmit an analogue signal requires, in principle, a perfect transmission path. In the case of an electrical voltage, any resistance in the transmission path will reduce the voltage at the receiving site. Analogue transmission, such as between the subscriber's house and the telephone exchange, is therefore susceptible to the introduction of noise. In contrast, the transmission of a digital signal is perfect. The huge advantage from the perspective of telemedicine is that transmission quality becomes independent of distance: a telemedicine transmission between two locations in the same city will work as well as transmission between two locations on different continents.

Box 2.3 Video standards

There are two common broadcast TV video standards: National Television Standards Committee (NTSC), which is used in Japan and North America, and Phase Alternating Line (PAL), which is used in much of Europe. The two systems have different display characteristics:

- 525 lines/picture at 30 pictures/s (NTSC),
- 625 lines/picture at 25 pictures/s (PAL).

The standard called common intermediate format (CIF), which is widely used for videoconferencing, was introduced to provide compatibility between the two video standards. Thus, it is possible to videoconference between the USA (where the camera and monitor operate to the NTSC standard) and say Europe (where the camera and monitor operate to the PAL standard). CIF is 288 lines/picture at 30 frames/s. The resulting quality of a CIF video picture is not very different from that of a normal TV picture.

Table 2.2 ITU protocols

Protocol	Purpose
H.320	The oldest of the multimedia communication protocols. Defines a videotelephone operating on ISDN
H.324	A newer protocol defining videotelephony for the standard telephone network (PSTN). Poorer-quality pictures result because of the restricted bandwidth of the PSTN compared with ISDN. Since H.324 can also be used on ISDN, it may supersede H.320 in due course
H.323	A newer protocol defining videotelephony for LANs and the Internet
T.120	A family of protocols to allow computer-supported cooperative working in conjunction with videotelephony

equipment from different manufacturers is interoperable, international standards have been defined by the International Telecommunication Union (ITU) (Table 2.2). Provided that each telemedicine site has a system embracing the proper standards, it is possible to conduct videoconferencing sessions between pieces of equipment supplied by different manufacturers. This applies not just to the basic transmission of video and audio, but also to additional features such as the control of cameras at the remote site, and the exchange of data between PCs that are being used in the videoconferencing session. Equipment that does not adhere to standards should be avoided.

Compression is a rapidly developing area of computing science, where the objective is to maximize the file compression and minimize the information loss.

Videoconferencing equipment

Videoconferencing has traditionally required equipment which was expensive to buy and to run, and was large and complicated to operate. At first it could be used only in fixed studio installations, but miniaturization made possible the development of the 'rollabout' unit, which could be moved between rooms within a building. The basis of the equipment is the CODEC (coder/decoder), which handles the compression of video pictures prior to transmission, and the decompression of the received pictures prior to display. Rollabout units are still widely used, particularly in business, and generally deliver high-quality video pictures (up to 2 Mbit/s transmission) on large display monitors with high-quality sound.

More recently, as the trend to miniaturization has continued, portable videoconferencing units have appeared, in which all the components except the display screen are integrated into a single unit. Such 'set-top' units require only connecting to a domestic TV to form a good-quality videoconferencing system (Figure 2.4).

Further technological development has resulted in the videoconferencing functions becoming available on a plug-in card for PCs. This means that an ordinary PC can be used as a personal 'desktop' videoconferencing workstation delivering reasonable quality video on a smaller screen and with generally lower-quality sound; nonetheless, these may be adequate for many purposes. It is also possible to use the PC's own processor to encode video for transmission, i.e. the PC operates as a software CODEC (Figure 2.5).

The merits of the different families of videoconferencing system are summarized in Table 2.3.

Much of the technology to capture the different types of information required in telemedicine will be available in any well-equipped modern office, but most telemedicine applications aim to provide services to poorly equipped remote sites that may not have even the most basic computer equipment. A major part of the overall cost of setting up a telemedicine system may be purchasing such straightforward items for the patient consultation end of the link.

Information transmission

All of the above relates to videoconferencing equipment using digital tele-communications. It is also possible to transmit video pictures using the ordinary telephone network, but, because a very high degree of image compression is required, the picture quality is rather poor.

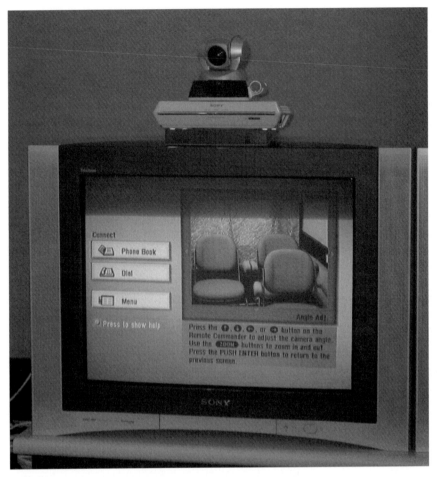

Figure 2.4 A set-top videoconferencing unit

In terms of network coverage, the conventional telephone is now widely available, even in the developing world; it is also a relatively inexpensive form of communication. More sophisticated digital telecommunications, such as ISDN, have more restricted coverage and higher costs, though they have major advantages over conventional telephony in terms of reliability and bandwidth. Satellite communications solve the coverage problem – providing truly global access – but remain expensive.

The choice of transmission method for any telemedicine application is, in practice, a compromise between what one would like and what one can afford. In practice, various trade-offs have to be made, which include:

- cost,
- availability of the service (i.e. the coverage),
- bandwidth, reliability and quality of service.

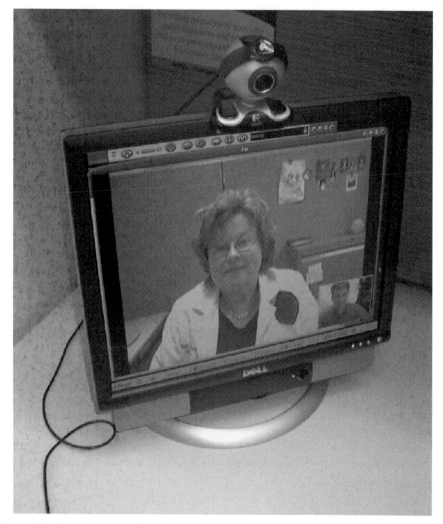

Figure 2.5 Desktop videoconferencing software (photo credit: B Harnett)

Table 2.3 Types of videoconferencing system

Type	Quality of video and audio	Cost	Usage
Studio	High	High	Large group
Rollabout	High	High	Small group
Set-top	Low/medium	Low	Personal/small group
Desktop	Low/medium	Low	Personal
PSTN	Low	Low	Personal

Cost

Telecommunications costs generally are falling. In most parts of the world, there is increased competition in the telecommunications industry, because of the privatization of previously government-run departments and deregulation. Another factor in falling prices is technological development. Nonetheless, telecommunications costs may still represent a significant proportion of the cost of a given telemedicine application.

Availability of the service

Despite the wide availability of network services, a common problem in telemedicine is the availability of network services over the 'last mile'. The 'last mile' describes the connection from the actual site of practice to the nearest telecommunication access point, such as the local telephone exchange. Providing a connection over this last mile is often where telecommunication becomes very expensive.

Bandwidth, reliability and quality of service

An important factor in telemedicine is the time frame in which the information is required. For some applications rapid information transfer is needed, for example when telemedicine is being performed for emergency management. However, in less urgent cases information can be stored and transmitted at a slower rate, for later examination.

Bandwidth is the data-carrying capacity of the communication medium used. It is measured in bits per second (bit/s, often abbreviated to bps) and ranges from 1200 bit/s for some types of mobile phones to more than 1000 Mbit/s for transmission through a fibre-optic cable. Successful telemedicine has been carried out using a wide range of bandwidths.

The clinical information to be transmitted will dictate the minimum network bandwidth that can be used.[11] How this bandwidth is obtained between the sites involved in the study depends on a variety of different factors. The main questions will be what infrastructure is already in place at each site, and what communications are possible between the sites (both physically and through local telecommunication companies). Rural areas where patients are often most in need of telemedicine services are often those where network communication may be limited. Providing high-bandwidth connections to such sites can be very expensive.

Generally speaking, the problems of network reliability (in the sense of communications being possible or not), exemplified by the traditional telephone network with electromechanical switching, have been solved by the move to digital telecommunications. In fact, substantial portions of the telephone network are already digital, which is partly why the call quality has improved dramatically over the last 20 years.

A related aspect to the general reliability of a telecommunications link is the quality of service that can be guaranteed for the user. For networks in which the user is provided with a circuit from end to end (such as ISDN or the PSTN) there is little difficulty, but for networks in which the bandwidth is shared (such as the Internet) the bandwidth available to the user can be severely affected by what other users are currently doing. In some networks with shared bandwidth, it is possible to reserve bandwidth for the user at the start of the connection and then release it to the general pool at the end. Such quality-of-service techniques have yet to be standardized.

The Internet

Most people are now familiar with modem access to the Internet via the telephone network, and this method of communication can be used for telemedicine.[12–15] Such systems have the advantage of accessibility, since anyone who can access the Internet can reach the required sites (*limiting* access to legitimate users may then be a problem, and security issues may become important). The Internet is particularly useful for situations where a clinician may require access to data from home (such as a radiologist viewing an X-ray image) before giving some clinical advice, e.g. a consultant advising on a fracture seen by a junior doctor in the emergency department. It may also be possible to use these systems from areas where analogue telephone lines are the only ones available, which may be particularly helpful for remote sites where other means of communication are limited.[16]

Web servers on the Internet store data for subsequent distribution to users. This is a client/server architecture, which is a useful approach for telemedicine. The Internet can also be used to provide a virtual private network (VPN), i.e. to provide a private (secure) connection between two sites. A VPN offers a method of securely linking sites. The limitation is that both sites must have connection to the Internet at the desired bandwidth. Many remote sites do not yet have Internet service providers (ISPs) with sufficient bandwidth available, although in cities this type of connection is worth considering. The alternative to a dial-on-demand connection is a dedicated or permanent circuit.

Standard telephony

The conventional telephone system is the public switched telephone network (PSTN). The standard analogue telephone line is a readily available form of communication, obtainable almost anywhere in the world. Unfortunately, the bandwidth available to users is limited to a maximum of 56 kbit/s and is likely to be much less if the telecommunications infrastructure is poor. Nonetheless, this type of connection can be suitable for some telemedicine applications that do not require either realtime data transmission or large file sizes. For applications such as teledermatology and telepathology, a modem connection may be sufficient to let two sites view images simultaneously, while discussing them via a separate telephone line.

Mobile phones

Mobile phones are becoming commonplace, and can be used to transmit digital data, albeit at low rates of data transfer (similar to the PTSN). For applications where realtime transfer is not needed and access to a standard modem is not possible, they are ideal. Mobile phones may be useful to connect with a specific individual who is travelling, and has access to a mobile phone and perhaps a laptop computer. Computerized tomography (CT) scans[17] and ECG recordings[18] have been reported in this way. This may be relevant in many developing nations, where mobile phone networks are being deployed instead of upgrading and expanding the traditional telephone network.

ISDN

The digital counterpart of the PSTN is ISDN, which is now available in most metropolitan areas in industrialized countries. It is completely different from the PSTN and offers end-to-end digital connectivity. This has two main advantages: greater reliability due to the digital nature of the data traffic, and higher bandwidth per line. Two standard types of ISDN connection are available to customers: a basic-rate line and a primary-rate line.

A basic-rate ISDN line offers the user a bandwidth of 128 kbit/s in two separate 64 kbit/s data channels. Basic-quality videoconferencing can be conducted using commercial equipment over a single basic-rate ISDN line. For higher-quality videoconferencing, multiple basic-rate ISDN lines can be used. For example, three lines aggregated together (providing six data channels) are commonly used, resulting in a bandwidth of 384 kbit/s. Primary-rate ISDN lines offer the user a bandwidth of up to 2 Mbit/s, thus allowing very high-quality video pictures to be transmitted.

ISDN connections are commonly used for telemedicine, because of their security, bandwidth, quality of service and relatively wide availability. Another advantage is the potential for adding capacity to these networks by renting additional lines. The major drawback of ISDN is that line rentals and usage charges can be high, although itemized billing allows the actual cost of telemedicine use to be readily evaluated.

A recent trend is to use existing local area networks (LANs) for telemedicine data transmission using Internet Protocol (IP). The principal disadvantage for realtime work is the problem of guaranteeing bandwidth for the telemedicine application.

Satellite

Generally speaking, fixed satellite connections are expensive to install and costly to use. They offer similar bandwidth to microwave links and the ISDN, but have the advantage of global coverage. Traditional satellite connections use geosynchronous satellites. Several telemedicine projects have used satellite linkages to connect mobile sites (such as military units or ships at sea) which would be impossible to reach in any other way.[19,20] As costs fall in the future, satellite transmission may become competitive with ISDN, particularly for remote areas. See Lamminen for a recent review.[21]

Another option is the use of a low earth orbiting satellite (LEOS). A LEOS offers the advantage of very inexpensive, hand-held receivers, not much larger than a standard mobile phone. They can be used nearly anywhere in the world, but currently have one significant drawback: very low data rates, of the order of 2.4–3.0 kbit/s. This may be acceptable if you need to send only a small file.

Leased lines

Leased lines are an alternative to using ISDN, in which a permanent digital connection is established between two locations. The user pays a fixed rental for the line, which includes the cost of all calls. The line is leased for an agreed term (usually annually) and is thus paid for regardless of use. In contrast, the cost of dial-on-demand services like the PSTN or ISDN depends on the actual usage of the circuit. Clearly, there will be a point at which a leased line becomes cheaper than a dial-on-demand connection, which will depend on the usage. However, the leased line option limits the user to transmission between the two locations that have been connected (e.g. two hospitals), unlike the use of ISDN, in which any other institution with an ISDN connection can be called, just as with a telephone.

Digital subscriber lines (DSL)

DSL technology, which is often referred to as 'broadband', provides an IP connection to the user. DSL connections come in a variety of types, such as symmetric and asymmetric – in the latter case, it is called ADSL. The generic acronym is xDSL. The important thing about DSL is that it uses the existing copper telephone wire that is usually already present in the facility. The main drawback is that the facility must be located within about 5 km of the telephone company's switch. ADSL usually provides more downstream bandwidth (i.e. to the user) than upstream. This is fine for downloading data, but is not necessarily suitable for realtime videoconferencing.

Cable modems

Cable TV is common in many metropolitan areas. The cable network represents a robust wiring system, which connects to homes and businesses. The same cable can be modified to act as a gateway to the Internet. Like xDSL, cable uses an inexpensive modem to provide more bandwidth than can be obtained with the PSTN. The principal drawback is that cable systems usually provide access through regional gateways, which means that if many people in a local area are using the service, the available bandwidth per user may decrease. Cable modems – like xDSL – also provide asymmetrical bandwidth to the user. However, their cost and bandwidth make cable and xDSL attractive options for low-cost telemedicine applications.

Microwave

Microwave connections are expensive to install, but inexpensive to maintain. The bandwidth available using microwave connections is high, 2–10 Mbit/s being common. However, microwave links are only feasible for sites that are relatively close together. Sites require direct line of sight to each other and must be less than about 30 km apart (less if the visibility is poor). For longer distances, repeater stations can be used, but the cost rapidly becomes prohibitive. The advantage of a microwave link is that there are virtually no running costs – the bandwidth is essentially free following installation. The disadvantage is that a microwave link connects just two locations, point to point.

ATM

ATM transmission was designed to take advantage of the characteristics of fibre-optic cables. Very high bandwidth transmission is therefore possible, the latest equipment operating at rates of gigabits per second. However, ATM is used primarily in the 'backbone' of a network. Thus, the major telecommunications carriers use ATM for long-haul transmission. While ATM has advantages in terms of capacity and quality of service, it is very uncommon for ATM to be directly connected at the user level, and few telemedicine applications have used ATM networks directly.

Network options for telemedicine are summarized in Table 2.4.

Information display

The method of information display will depend mainly on the format in which the information is originally captured. For example, audio information will usually be 'displayed' in the form of sound. Several options are available for displaying images. Videoconferencing units commonly use standard TV sets as their display, while still images are often displayed on PC monitors. However, PC monitors are sometimes used instead of TV screens for viewing video, and TV screens are sometimes used for viewing the output from a PC. This is more than a matter of simply connecting them together, because PC display monitors and TV screens operate in a fundamentally different way (see Squibb for a review).[22]

Many items of medical equipment have a PC built-in, the output of which can be directly displayed on another PC but not viewed with a TV. In such cases, it may be necessary to use a specific video output (often designed for connection to a video recorder) to acquire an analogue signal suitable for a TV display. Such PCs do not always use bulky cathode ray tubes, but increasingly use flat screen displays (as in laptop computers). These types of display are still expensive, but are becoming increasingly popular due to their smaller overall size and lower power consumption. PC screens also come with different resolutions (the number of dots per unit area). High-resolution screens are used for detailed work, but are more expensive. Most telemedicine applications (other than radiology and pathology studies) do not need high-definition images. For instance, a standard magnetic resonance image (MRI) has a resolution of 512×512 pixels.

Table 2.4 Options for telecommunications

System	Typical data transfer rate	Coverage	Running costs	Capital costs	Uses	Advantages/disadvantages
PSTN	33.6–56 kbit/s	Ubiquitous	Low	Low	Data (e.g. text reports)	Inexpensive, available everywhere but slow and limited to simple data
Mobile phone	19.2–100 kbit/s +	Commonly available in industrialized countries	Low	Low (for the user, not necessarily for the provider)	Data (e.g. text reports)	Highly portable, easy to use; can have radio interference problems
Cable modems	>1 Mbit/s downstream; 2–300 upstream	Commonly available in industrialized countries	Low	Low	Data, images, limited video	Bandwidth is shared in local areas; asymmetrical
xDSL	>1 Mbit/s downstream; 2–300 upstream	Commonly available in industrialized countries	Low	Low	Data, images, limited video	Bandwidth is limited based on distance from telephone company's switch; asymmetrical
ISDN (basic rate)	128 kbit/s	Commonly available in industrialized countries	Medium	Low	Data (text, still images); some video (e.g. telepsychiatry)	Inexpensive but slow and not available everywhere
ISDN (primary rate)	1.54 or 2 Mbit/s	Commonly available in industrialized countries	High	High	Any (e.g. motion video tele-ultrasound)	Very flexible and high quality; expensive and not available everywhere
Leased lines	64 kbit/s–2 Mbit/s +	Available in many countries	Low/medium	High	Any	Inflexible, expensive to set up; large number of telemedicine episodes required before cost-effectiveness achieved
Microwave	<30 Mbit/s	Available in many countries	Very low	High	Any	High quality; localized and can be used only over short distances
Satellite	64 kbit/s–2 Mbit/s +	Global coverage	High	High	Any	High quality, high cost but can reach really remote areas
ATM	155 Mbit/s and up	Restricted use	Medium–high	High	Any	Very high bandwidth; used primarily as a network backbone

Training

Equipment and the telecommunications are a necessary, but not sufficient, prerequisite for a successful telemedicine programme. The right people are also required and they must be properly trained. Since many telemedicine programmes often begin incrementally, training users can also be done incrementally. Numerous universities and private companies offer telemedicine training, as well as the equipment vendors, although this sort of training tends to focus on the capabilities of specific devices. If you decide to implement a telemedicine programme, training must be part of the plan.

Conclusion

About 10 or 15 years ago, the technology for telemedicine was not readily available. Much early telemedicine work involved modification of expensive equipment, which was originally designed for other purposes. Now, however, the technologies such as robust telecommunication networks and video equipment are widely available, and much more affordable. Telemedicine users now have a plethora of choice. Most manufacturers offer products that adhere to industry standards which ensure interoperability with other devices. The situation in medical informatics is less developed and efforts continue to ensure the seamless integration of data between different systems. This is important in health care, where patient data-sets need to be available when required.

While the right technology is necessary for a successful telemedicine programme, it is essential not to overlook the human factors. In particular, a local 'champion' will be required, and there will be a continuing requirement for user training.

References

1   Hailey D, Ohinmaa A, Roine R. Study quality and evidence of benefit in recent assessments of telemedicine. *J Telemed Telecare* 2004;**10**:318–24
2   Mair F, Whitten P. Systematic review of studies of patient satisfaction with telemedicine. *BMJ* 2000;**320**:1517–20
3   High WA, Houston MS, Calobrisi SD, Drage LA, McEvoy MT. Assessment of the accuracy of low-cost store-and-forward teledermatology consultation. *J Am Acad Dermatol* 2000;**42**:776–83
4   Hoijtink EJ, Rascher I. Telemedicine training & treatment centre 'a European rollout of a medical best practice'. *Stud Health Technol Inform* 2005;**114**:270–3
5   Garfield MJ, Watson RT. Four case studies in state-supported telemedicine initiatives. *Telemed J E Health* 2003;**9**:197–205
6   McLendon K. Electronic medical record systems as a basis for computer-based patient records. *J AHIMA* 1993;**64**:50, 52, 54–5
7   Schadow G, Russler DC, Mead CN, McDonald CJ. Integrating medical information and knowledge in the HL7 RIM. *Proc AMIA Symp* 2000;764–8
8   Taylor P. A survey of research in telemedicine. 1: Telemedicine systems. *J Telemed Telecare* 1998;**4**:1–17

9   Vassallo DJ. Twelve months' experience with telemedicine for the British armed forces. *J Telemed Telecare* 1999;**5**:117–18

10   Lian P, Chong K, Zhai X, Ning Y. The quality of medical records in teleconsultation. *J Telemed Telecare* 2003;**9**:35–41

11   Rosser Jr JC, Bell RL, Harnett B, Rodas E, Murayama M, Merrell R. Use of mobile low-bandwidth telemedical techniques for extreme telemedicine applications. *J Am Coll Surg* 1999;**189**:397–404

12   Della Mea V, Puglisi F, Forti S, *et al*. Expert pathology consultation through the Internet: melanoma versus benign melanocytic tumours. *J Telemed Telecare* 1997;**3**:17–19

13   Kirby B, Lyon CC, Harrison PV. Low-cost teledermatology using Internet image transmission. *J Telemed Telecare* 1998;**4**:107

14   Johnson DS, Goel RP, Birtwistle P, Hirst P. Transferring medical images on the World Wide Web for emergency clinical management: a case report. *BMJ* 1998;**316**:988–9

15   Stålberg E, Stålberg S. Regional network in clinical neurophysiology, tele-EMG. In: Wootton R, ed. *European Telemedicine 1998/99*. London: Kensington Publications, 1999:101–3

16   Samedov RN. An Internet station for telemedicine in the Azerbaijan Republic. *J Telemed Telecare* 1998;**4**:42–3

17   Reponen J, Ilkko E, Jyrkinen L, *et al*. Digital wireless radiology consultations with a portable computer. *J Telemed Telecare* 1998;**4**:201–5

18   Freedman SB. Direct transmission of electrocardiograms to a mobile phone for management of a patient with acute myocardial infarction. *J Telemed Telecare* 1999;**5**:67–9

19   Paul NL. Telepsychiatry, the satellite system and family consultation. *J Telemed Telecare* 1997;**3**:52–3

20   Macedonia CR, Littlefield RJ, Coleman J, *et al*. Three-dimensional ultrasonographic telepresence. *J Telemed Telecare* 1998;**4**:224–30

21   Lamminen H. Mobile satellite systems. *J Telemed Telecare* 1999;**5**:71–83

22   Squibb NJ. Video transmission for telemedicine. *J Telemed Telecare* 1999;**5**:1–10

Further information

1   Maheu MM, Allen A, Whitten P. *E-Health, Telehealth, and Telemedicine: A Guide to Start-up and Success*. San Francisco: Jossey-Bass, 2001

2   Dodd AZ. *The Essential Guide to Telecommunications*. Upper Saddle River, NJ: Prentice Hall PTR, 1999

3   Radiological Society of North America. *A Non-Technical Introduction to DICOM*. See http://www.rsna.org/practice/dicom/intro/ (last checked 1 February 2005)

Section 2: Telemedicine Applications

▶3

Prerecorded telemedicine

Vincenzo Della Mea

Introduction

Prerecorded telemedicine is that form of telemedicine where the information being exchanged between the two sites is recorded (stored) in some format, either before or after it is transmitted. The point about this is that the person sending the information and the person receiving it do not need to do so simultaneously; thus, viewing the information can be done at some later time. Such systems are also called *store-and-forward* systems, as this indicates two of the principal steps involved in performing this type of telemedicine.

Prerecorded telemedicine is by no means new and has formed an integral part of much medical activity for many years. In fact, every time diagnostic materials such as radiographs, pathology glass slides or printed electrocardiographic recordings are sent by post to a colleague for a second opinion, or sent to an expert for a specialist opinion, a prerecorded telemedicine episode could be said to have occurred. Nowadays, however, prerecorded telemedicine can be performed in many more ways. Diagnosis and clinical management are the principal applications of prerecorded telemedicine and are the main focus of this chapter, although quality control and education, discussed in Chapter 5, are increasingly being performed using prerecorded telemedicine.

When to use prerecorded telemedicine

Prerecorded telemedicine is not appropriate for emergency consultations, since by definition there will be a delay before a response is received. Prerecorded telemedicine should be used only for non-urgent work, and in cases where all the information required to conduct a satisfactory episode can be acquired without any intervention on the part of the person receiving it. There are two main ways this can be performed.

(1) All the information is acquired and then transmitted. This is particularly suitable for those medical procedures where normal practice is to record everything. One of the main problems with this approach, however, is that so much data can be generated that it becomes impractical to store and transmit the information.

(2) All the information is acquired, but the sender then reviews it and forwards only that which is considered relevant or necessary. This is known as sampling and results in the need for less storage space and quicker transmission of information.

Information sampling introduces its own problems, however. The main one is that such an approach assumes that the sender of the information has the skill and training to be able to decide what information is necessary and what can be discarded. This has implications regarding responsibility and liability because the expert will not have all of the crude information available. If sampling at the sender's site is not an option, an alternative is to reduce the amount of information using data compression techniques (discussed in Chapter 2), or for the expert at the receiving end to perform the sampling. This latter approach, however, involves realtime interaction; such techniques are discussed in Chapter 4. The following examples illustrate some of the problems encountered when performing prerecorded telemedicine.

Store-and-forward telepathology

Pathology is an image-based discipline in which a diagnosis is made by examining the visually perceptible features of lesions. The images are obtained in many ways, one of which is viewing cut specimens of the lesion that have been fixed on glass slides, using a light microscope. During examination of the specimens, a pathologist will view one or more glass slides through a microscope, at up to six different magnifications. A large part of the examination is therefore screening to locate interesting fields or abnormal areas. This process if replicated in full would generate a colossal amount of information that would not be easily manageable. Thus, the quantity of information acquired needs to be reduced before it is transmitted. This is done either by compression techniques or by the sender sampling the slides and forwarding only those areas that are felt to be of diagnostic significance. Such an approach permits the amount of data for transmission to be reduced to just hundreds of kBytes, making store-and-forward transmission technically feasible.

Ultrasonography

During ultrasonography, a transducer is moved over the area to be examined, producing a continuous stream of low-resolution video pictures. As in pathology, if all these video images were to be recorded, a huge amount of information would be generated, much of which would be of no diagnostic value. The long-established practice of taking still photographs from the continuous video closely resembles the sampling that occurs in prerecorded telemedicine.

Assuming that the above requirements can be met, prerecorded telemedicine should always be considered before realtime telemedicine. This is because it is less trouble to organize, as it is not necessary for all parties to be involved simultaneously. Lower-bandwidth connections between less sophisticated systems will also suffice, resulting in lower operating costs. Against these benefits, however, it may not be possible to provide an immediate result in a prerecorded telemedicine episode, and there is potentially less of an educational component than in realtime telemedicine interactions.

Technical aspects of prerecorded telemedicine

In prerecorded telemedicine systems, the following steps can be distinguished:

(1) the acquisition of diagnostic information at the remote site;
(2) its storage, which can be at either site, or at both;
(3) its delivery to the expert site through an appropriate connection;
(4) its display at the expert site.

These steps are outlined in Figure 3.1. After analysis of the information, the prerecorded telemedicine process may be reversed by transmitting the results of any episode back to the remote site. Alternatively, any communication could be done in realtime, for example using the telephone, at which time the expert could discuss his or her findings with someone at the remote site.

Information acquisition

As described in Chapter 2, many different types of clinical information can be transmitted between sites using telemedicine, and some of these are more suited than others to prerecorded telemedicine. How information can be captured and in what format has been discussed already. For information which is generated at source in digital form, such as digital radiography, PACS (picture archive and communication system), MRI, CT scanners and digital cameras, no conversion is required. However, for other modalities, such as conventional film-based radiographs, analogue video cameras, sonography and ECG recordings on paper, digitization of the information is necessary.

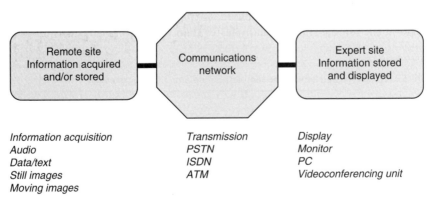

Figure 3.1 Steps in a prerecorded telemedicine system

Compression and storage issues

For many prerecorded telemedicine applications, the quantity of information is often very large. As transmission time depends on the quantity of information being transmitted (file size), methods for reducing the amount of storage required in prerecorded telemedicine are usually necessary. The main way to achieve this is to apply some kind of a compression algorithm, as discussed in Chapter 2. In summary, these are of two kinds: either lossless (i.e. completely reversible) or lossy (i.e. with a loss of information, so that a compressed and then decompressed file is different from the original one). Lossless methods produce compression ratios of up to 1:3, while lossy methods are more efficient, with selectable levels of compression (which could be up to 100–200:1). The most well known lossy algorithm for images is that of the Joint Photographic Experts Group (JPEG). Table 3.1 shows some typical storage sizes in different telemedicine applications, with compressed file sizes at common compression ratios.

Storage in itself does not create any new problems in prerecorded telemedicine, except when the files are extremely large. One important issue that is often neglected, however, involves file formats. In order to maximize the exchange of information between as many sites as possible, some standard should be adopted. Note that storage in prerecorded telemedicine does not always require the use of computers; for example, video images are sometimes recorded onto VHS tape and then delivered by post for expert interpretation.

Transmission

Once the information has been acquired and stored, it can then be transmitted. How quickly this can be achieved depends on the quantity of information and the network used. Figure 3.2 shows the time needed to send a 2 MByte data-set at different bandwidths, corresponding to modems on conventional telephone lines (at 57.6 kbit/s), a basic-rate ISDN line (128 kbit/s), three ISDN lines used together (384 kbit/s), a typical ADSL upload rate (512 kbit/s), a primary-rate ISDN line (2 Mbit/s), and finally an Ethernet network running at 10 and 100 Mbit/s.

It should be noted that ADSL connections usually have asymmetric bandwidths for download and upload; in particular, download (i.e. reception of data at the remote site) is usually faster than upload (i.e. transmission of data

Table 3.1 Some typical telemedicine samples, before and after compression

Data type	Dimensions	Bit/sample	File size (MByte)	File size after compression (kByte)	Compression ratio
Radiograph	2000 × 2000 pixels	12	5.7	285	20:1
Pathology microscope image	800 × 600 pixels	24 (8 × 3)	1.44	96	15:1
CT data-set (20 images)	256 × 256 pixels per image	8	1.3	650	2:1
Dermatology image	1280 × 1024 pixels	24 (8 × 3)	3.9	980	4:1
20 s heart sound	441,000 samples	16	0.882	440	2:1
10 s, 12-lead ECG	5000 × 12 samples	12	0.090	45	2:1

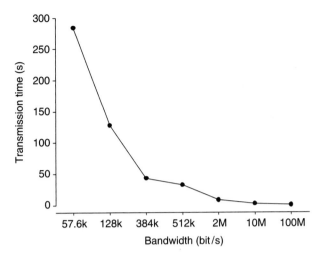

Figure 3.2 Time needed to send a 2 MByte file

from the remote site). This should be taken into account when evaluating the use of ADSL for telemedicine.

There are three principal models for how transmission is performed in prerecorded telemedicine:

(1) direct communication between the sites;
(2) using a central server as a broker;
(3) using a generalized server infrastructure.

Direct communication

With direct communication there is a direct link between the sites (Figure 3.3). This may be a dial-on-demand link using the existing telecommunications infrastructure or a dedicated connection. The main advantage of direct links is greater privacy, and hence patient confidentiality is more likely to be protected. The main disadvantage is that there is a need for the sites to be operational at all times. This may be a particular problem if the distances involved are great and the sites are located in different time zones.

Using a central server as a broker

A practical way for overcoming the main limitation of direct links between the sites is to make use of a server (Figure 3.4). In this approach, the sender transmits the acquired medical data to the server, on a specific communication channel. The recipient can then receive or download the information from the server at a convenient time. In addition, the server can receive information from more than one sender and can actively process the information transmitted to it, allowing benefits such as archiving cases for long-term storage for medicolegal purposes.

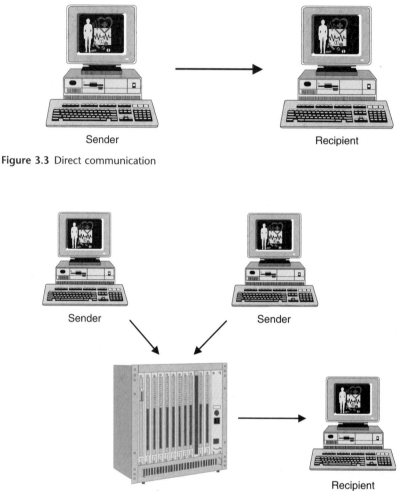

Figure 3.3 Direct communication

Figure 3.4 Server-mediated communication – central server acting as an information broker

A disadvantage of such a system, however, is that its performance reduces as the number of telemedicine episodes increases.

Using a generalized server infrastructure

A generalization of the above approach is to link several servers, each one of which supports a group of users, on either a geographical or an institutional basis (Figure 3.5). A sender is then able to transmit information to the local server which, because it is linked with other servers, can forward the information to other sites, which may or may not be within the locality of the sender. Such a model, which in fact is the basic model used for electronic mail on the Internet,

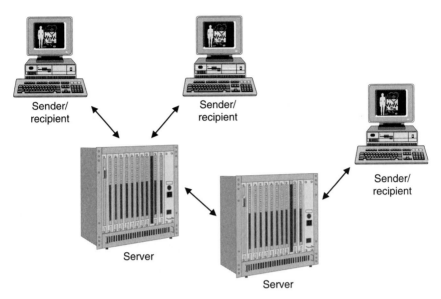

Figure 3.5 Multi-server communication – generalized server infrastructure

shares the workload between different severs, and permits access by many other users.

A more complicated version of the generalized server infrastructure is the so-called peer-to-peer paradigm, where data can be distributed over a number of nodes of a network.

Information display

The display of information obtained through prerecorded telemedicine systems follows the criteria presented in Chapter 2.

Types of prerecorded telemedicine

The types of information transferred may be used to categorize the different kinds of prerecorded telemedicine:

- audio;
- data and text;
- still images;
- moving images (i.e. video).

So far most work in prerecorded telemedicine has been done with data and text, and with still images. Video is increasingly being transmitted for tele-medicine. Examples of each category are considered below.

Transfer of prerecorded audio

Prerecorded transfer of audio includes the transmission of heart sounds. For example, the Department of Paediatrics at the University of Tromsø in Norway is linked to two health centres. This permits a general practitioner who hears a suspicious heart murmur to record the patient's heart sounds with a digital stethoscope, add the recording to a referral letter and send it by email to a specialist for evaluation.[1] Desktop PCs fitted with a sound card and a network connection are used.

Transfer of prerecorded data and text

Data can be transferred using the ordinary telephone network by a modem, by fax, by Internet communications, or by mobile phone.

Tele-ECG

The ECG represents the electrical activity of the heart and is particularly suitable for store-and-forward telemedicine from a technical point of view. In prerecorded electrocardiography, an ECG device with internal storage (usually available in portable units) records the electrical signals, which are usually sampled from a number of leads. The digitized data are then transmitted to a workstation, from where the signal can be displayed on a video monitor or printed. Transmission of signals usually occurs through telephone-based digital links,[2] either fixed or mobile, although the simple transmission by fax of scanned images of the printed ECGs has also proved successful.[3]

Tele-EEG

The electroencephalogram (EEG) represents the electrical activity of the brain and consists of multiple channels (up to 32) of brain wave patterns. The EEG examination is suitable for modern telemedicine applications because the data are either produced in, or can easily be converted to, digital form. The duration of routine EEG recordings varies from 15 to 60 min. When digitized, EEGs result in large files; for example, a 30 min, 32-channel digital EEG recording digitized at a sampling rate of 200 Hz and 16 bits results in a file size of 23 MByte. Using a 57.6 kbit/s modem on the telephone network would require a transmission time of more than 50 min.

Several tele-EEG programmes have been operational since the mid-1960s in various parts of the world. One of these programmes, pioneered by Professor Max House in the late 1970s at the Memorial University Hospital of Newfoundland, has dealt with over 10,000 EEG recordings.[4] Such are the levels of activity of tele-EEG that the American Electroencephalographic Society has drawn up guidelines for the telephone transmission of EEGs.[5]

Tele-neurophysiology

Clinical neurophysiology is a specialty related to physiological studies of the central and peripheral nervous system. The central nervous system is investigated with tests such as the EEG and visual evoked potentials, while the peripheral nervous system is investigated with electromyography and nerve conduction studies. The data generated by these tests are increasingly in digital form. Several regional networks in clinical neurophysiology have been established. In Uppsala, Sweden, the central laboratory serves nine satellite sites, with data being transmitted via modem to the main laboratory, Internet communication being used for some of the files. Connections with more distant laboratories are also in place for second opinions and for collaboration for collection of reference values.[6]

Tele-ophthalmology

Ophthalmology is the study of diseases of the eye and the orbit. Prerecorded data and text transfer in ophthalmology are mainly used for electrodiagnostic purposes. For example, the Electrodiagnostic Neurophysiological Automated Analysis telematic system provides facilities for tests such as electroretinography, electro-oculography and pattern-reversal visual evoked potentials. In all, 4500 electrodiagnostic tests, administered to 130 normal subjects and 1000 patients in five laboratories in three European countries and one laboratory in an Asian country, have been transmitted to the Bristol Eye Hospital in the UK. The results from both the normal subjects and the patients show that ophthalmic electro-diagnosis is possible using telemedicine.[7]

Tele-obstetrics

Pre-term births and late fetal deaths are important causes of perinatal morbidity and mortality. The idea of monitoring uterine contractions as a means of predicting those pregnancies at risk of pre-term labour arose in the late 1970s. In Hungary, telemedical home monitoring of such activity, with transmission to the obstetrician's PC via an ordinary telephone line, has been shown to be feasible and to result in a halving of the pre-term birth rate in the monitored pregnancies.[8]

Patient–physician electronic mail communication

In principle, prerecorded telemedicine would be useful for patient and doctor communication, i.e. email messages used for diagnostic or therapeutic purposes. This application is growing more slowly than one might expect, partly because of fears that doctors will become overloaded with email correspondence, and partly because of concerns about security and privacy when messages are sent over the public Internet.

Transfer of prerecorded still images

The most widely used application in prerecorded telemedicine is teleradiology. Other examples are also described below.

Teleradiology

One of the most mature applications in telemedicine is teleradiology, which can be defined as the electronic transmission of radiological images from one site to another. It has a longer history than most other telemedicine applications; for example, dental radiographs were sent by telegraph as early as 1929. Many different types of radiological images can be transmitted, including radiographs, CT scans and MRI scans. Telemammography involves the transmission of very-high-resolution images, and is the most recently developed telemedicine technique in this field.[9]

The rapid growth in teleradiology usage has resulted in a series of standards and guidelines for its proper use in certain situations.[10] Ruggiero has reviewed the subject.[11]

Telepathology

The development of prerecorded telepathology has been hindered because of unresolved issues surrounding the sampling of images before their transmission for expert interpretation. However, the recent publishing of a study by the Armed Forces Institute of Pathology (AFIP) regarding 1255 second-consultation telepathology cases helped to clarify the performance of prerecorded telepathology[12] (with 97% agreement versus diagnosis at the microscope). The AFIP is one of the two institutions where telepathology consultations can be obtained, together with the Telepathology Consultation Centre of the International Union Against the Cancer.

Furthermore, a novel technique has been developed, called the 'digital' or 'virtual' slide, which allows the recording of a complete digital slide, resulting in hundreds of MBytes of data.[13] By accessing such a data-set, the sampling problem is solved. For its transmission, two techniques are available: transfer of the complete data-set (preferably overnight, due to the size), or access through a software program (often called a virtual microscope) able to transfer on demand just the images requested by the user.

Teledermatology

Prerecorded teledermatology involves capturing one or more images of a dermatological condition and then forwarding them to a specialist, together with other relevant clinical information for interpretation. The images can be still or moving pictures. It can be as simple as sending a photograph of a lesion in the post to a specialist, or it can involve transmitting a prerecorded digital image to the specialist via a high-speed communications network. The main use of teledermatology is remote consultation, either between primary and secondary care (e.g. a general practitioner asking advice from a hospital dermatologist) or between dermatologists.

The levels of diagnostic agreement between teledermatology consultations and face-to-face consultations have been found to be between 51% and 95% in different studies. This is similar to levels of inter-observer agreement between dermatologists examining patients face to face.[14]

Tele-ophthalmology

Recent developments in digital photography offer new and exciting possibilities in the detection, assessment and management of diseases of the eye.[15] One condition of interest, which is the leading cause of blindness in the young adult population in the Western world, is diabetes mellitus. Digital technology permits better storage and retrieval facilities, and image enhancement for improved detection and analysis. Such images are more and more used for the screening and management of diabetic patients.[16]

Transfer of prerecorded moving images (video)

There are fewer examples of prerecorded moving images being transferred compared with static images, due to their larger file size. Examples of projects that have been performed include intravascular ultrasound video images,[17] and the improvement of asthma outcome in children by Internet transmission and examination of videos of peak flow meter use.[18]

Prerecorded telemedicine using email

An increasingly common way of doing prerecorded telemedicine is by email sent via the Internet. Although there are some problems associated with the Internet, its wide availability and low cost have encouraged those interested in telemedicine to evaluate its usefulness.[19] Examples where email has been used successfully include:

- teleradiology;[20]
- telecardiology;[21]
- teledermatology;[22]
- telepathology.[23]

Prerecorded telemedicine using email may use special-purpose software, such as TeleMedMail, on the referrer's computer to construct the referral message.[24] This has the advantage that all the relevant information is likely to be included (Figure 3.6). However, the disadvantage is the necessity to load special software onto the referrer's computer. Successful telemedicine is also possible using ordinary Internet email.[25]

Conclusion

In some situations prerecorded telemedicine is the only way to provide remote medical services. In other instances, it is the most cost-effective method and associated with the least organizational upset. For example, because transmission and ultimately display occur at a time different from that of data acquisition, there is no need for all parties to be present simultaneously. Data archiving can also be added easily to a prerecorded telemedicine system and this may have certain medicolegal advantages. Clearly, however, there are also situations when prerecorded telemedicine is not an appropriate way to deliver health services; for example, whenever the sender of the information is not qualified to sample the

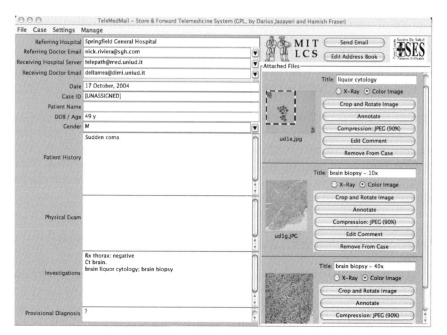

Figure 3.6 A TeleMedMail screenshot

information acquired or the specialist receiving the information must manipulate it, during acquisition, in some way.

The increasing interest in low-cost telemedicine has shifted attention from relatively expensive realtime, high-bandwidth systems to more affordable prerecorded methods. Email is a particularly attractive option in this regard because of its cheapness and ubiquity. In the past, the ever-increasing use of email in health-care delivery, including email usage among medical professionals, suggested a future where many telemedicine consultations would be conducted using secure multimedia email messages. However, in the last few years, this prospect has been undermined by, for example, the large quantities of unsolicited email ('spam') and viruses. This may be one reason for the switch towards Web-based telemedicine services, which offer almost the same features as email, but depend on a different infrastructure. An example of such services is the iPath software suite, which allows for the delivery of store-and-forward telemedicine cases to a Web server, where discussions about the cases may occur in a semi-interactive way.[26]

References

1   Elford DR. Telemedicine in northern Norway. *J Telemed Telecare* 1997;**3**:1–22
2   Ducasse R, Hardman DD. Transtelephonic cardiac monitoring: a comprehensive review of clinical applications. *Crit Care Nurse* 1988;**8**:44–51

3   Ong K, Chia P, Ng WL, Choo M. A telemedicine system for high-quality transmission of paper electrocardiographic reports. *J Telemed Telecare* 1995;**1**:27–33

4   House AM, Roberts JM. Telemedicine in Canada. *Canad Med Assoc J* 1977;**117**:386–8

5   American Electroencephalographic Society. Guideline six: recommendations for telephone transmission of EEGs. *J Clin Neurophysiol* 1994;**11**:28–9

6   Stålberg E, Stålberg S. Regional network in clinical neurophysiology, tele-EMG. In: Wootton R, ed. *European Telemedicine 1998/99*. London: Kensington Publications, 1999:101–3

7   Papakostopoulos D, Hart JC, Papakostopoulos S, Dodson K, Williams A. Standardized visual evoked potentials for telematic electrodiagnosis from five laboratories in three European countries. *J Telemed Telecare* 1999;**5**:23–31

8   Torok M, Turi Z, Kovacs F. Ten years' clinical experience with telemedicine in prenatal care in Hungary. *J Telemed Telecare* 1999;**5** (Suppl. 1):14–17

9   James JJ. The current status of digital mammography. *Clin Radiol* 2004;**59**:1–10

10   De Moor GJE, Van Maele G, eds. *Standards in Health Care Informatics and Telematics*. European Committee for Standardisation – Technical Committee 251: Medical Informatics, 1996

11   Ruggiero C. Teleradiology: a review. *J Telemed Telecare* 1998;**4**:25–35

12   Williams BH, Mullick FG, Butler DR, Herring RF, O'Leary TJ. Clinical evaluation of an international static image-based telepathology service. *Hum Pathol* 2001;**32**:1309–1317

13   Demichelis F, Barbareschi M, Dalla Palma P, Forti S. The virtual case: a new method to completely digitize cytological and histological slides. *Virchows Arch* 2002;**441**:159–164

14   Whited JD. Teledermatology. Current status and future directions. *Am J Clin Dermatol* 2001;**2**:59–64

15   Taylor P, Kennedy C, Murdoch I, Johnston K, Cook C, Godoumov R. Assessment of benefit in tele-ophthalmology using a consensus panel. *J Telemed Telecare* 2003;**9**:140–5

16   Choremis J, Chow DR. Use of telemedicine in screening for diabetic retinopathy. *Canad J Ophthalmol* 2003;**38**:575–9

17   Stahl JN, Zhang J, Zellner C, Pomerantsev EV, Chou TN, Huang HK. A new approach to teleconferencing with intravascular US and cardiac angiography in a low-bandwidth environment. *Radiographics* 2000;**20**:1495–503

18   Chan DS, Callahan CW, Sheets SJ, Moreno CN, Malone FJ. An Internet-based store-and-forward video home telehealth system for improving asthma outcomes in children. *Am J Health-Syst Pharm* 2003;**60**:1976–81

19   Della Mea V. Internet electronic mail: a tool for low-cost telemedicine. *J Telemed Telecare* 1999;**5**:84–9

20   Szot A, Jacobson FL, Munn S, *et al*. Diagnostic accuracy of chest X-rays acquired using a digital camera for low-cost teleradiology. *Int J Med Inform* 2004;**73**:65–73

21   Tually P, Janssen J, Cowell S, Walker J. A preliminary assessment of Internet-based nuclear telecardiology to support the clinical management of cardiac disease in a remote community. *J Telemed Telecare* 2003;**9** (Suppl. 1):69–71

22   van den Akker TW, Reker CH, Knol A, Post J, Wilbrink J, van der Veen JP. Teledermatology as a tool for communication between general practitioners and dermatologists. *J Telemed Telecare* 2001;**7**:193–8

23   Della Mea V, Beltrami CA. Telepathology applications of the Internet multimedia electronic mail. *Med Inform* 1998;**23**:237–44

24   Fraser HS, Jazayeri D, Bannach L, Szolovits P, McGrath SJ. TeleMedMail: free software to facilitate telemedicine in developing countries. *Medinfo* 2001;**10**:815–19

25   Wootton R, Youngberry K, Swinfen P, Swinfen R. Prospective review of a global e-health system for doctors in developing countries. *J Telemed Telecare* 2004;**10** (Suppl. 1):94–6

26   Brauchli K, Christen H, Meyer P, *et al*. Telepathology: design of a modular system. *Anal Cell Pathol* 2000;**21**:193–9

Further information

1   Kane B, Sands DZ. Guidelines for the clinical use of electronic mail with patients. The AMIA Internet Working Group, Task Force on Guidelines for the Use of Clinic–Patient Electronic Mail. *J Am Med Inform Assoc* 1998;**5**:104–111. Available at http://www.pubmedcentral.nih.gov/articlerender.fcgi?tool=pubmed&pubmedid=9452989I (last checked 30 December 2004)

2   Teledermatology Special Interest Group of the American Telemedicine Association. *Protocols and Guides for Store-and-Forward Teledermatology*. See http://www.atmeda.org/ICOT/sigtelederm.htm (last checked 10 November 2004)

3   Telepathology Consultation Center of the Union Internationale Contre le Cancer (UICC). An example of an institutional, not-for-profit teleconsultation centre, which uses store-and-forward telemedicine via a web server. See http://pathoweb.charite.de/UICC-TPCC/ (last checked 10 November 2004)

4   Swinfen Charitable Trust. A global, not-for-profit e-referral network for doctors in hospitals in developing countries. The system is based on the use of ordinary Internet email. See http://www.uq.edu.au/swinfen (last checked 10 November 2004)

▶4

Realtime telemedicine

Richard Wootton

Introduction

Telemedicine is about the transmission of information. Very often this information is provided to satisfy a specific request (e.g. in diagnosis or clinical management), but it may be more general information (e.g. in education). Distance education is considered in detail in Chapter 5. This chapter focuses on realtime telemedicine for diagnosis and clinical management.

There are two fundamentally different ways of providing the information in a telemedicine 'event'. The information may be provided in realtime, with all parties – even if not physically present in the same location – being able to interact at once; a telephone conversation is an example of a realtime interaction. Alternatively, the information may be provided for examination by the party being consulted at some later time, i.e. it is prerecorded. This is often called a 'store-and-forward' technique, and although the term is not always strictly accurate it has become commonplace. An email message is an example of such a technique.

The terms synchronous and asynchronous are also sometimes used to describe realtime and prerecorded transmissions, based on the idea of virtual meeting of the parties involved.

Although telemedicine is commonly thought to be a recent phenomenon, its history is much older than 20th-century medicine, and certainly goes back to pre-electronic days (see Chapter 1). However, it is the availability of low-cost digital computing and communication in the last 10–20 years that has triggered the growth in telemedicine. Recent surveys[1] show that much current telemedicine activity involves realtime telemedicine, although a substantial proportion is prerecorded.

When to use realtime telemedicine

There is no doubt that telemedicine conducted via prerecorded interaction is more convenient than that using realtime interaction: it is not necessary to arrange a simultaneous meeting between 'client' and 'expert'. Furthermore, a lower-bandwidth connection will usually suffice (e.g. the Internet), which will be cheaper, as will the equipment required at each end.

Table 4.1 Advantages of types of telemedicine

Prerecorded	Realtime
More convenient – no need for simultaneous meetings to be arranged	Immediate result. Also the specialist can request any missing information immediately
Low-bandwidth interaction – cheaper telecommunications; cheaper equipment	Meets consumer expectations – patients like the three-way consultation
	Educational benefit

On the other hand, a realtime consultation allows an immediate result to be obtained. If the expert requires additional information from the client, it can be provided immediately. The delays intrinsic to the use of email, for example, are avoided. In addition, the realtime interaction between client and expert contains a strong educational component. As well as (one hopes) providing an answer to the immediate query, there is an element of continuing medical education in the encounter, if not at first consultation, then certainly as consultations continue over time. This educational benefit of realtime telemedicine is hard to quantify, but has been reported by several well established programmes. Bergmo estimated that a rural general practitioner engaged in weekly tele-ENT (ear, nose and throat) clinics in northern Norway was able to reduce his referral rate by 50% after the first year, as a result of his improved knowledge, obtained through interacting with the specialist.[2] Table 4.1 summarizes the advantages of realtime telemedicine.

When should realtime telemedicine be preferred to prerecorded telemedicine? Clearly, when the importance of an immediate result outweighs the disadvantages of inconvenience and cost. For example, if a teleconsultation was required for a life-threatening injury, a store-and-forward interaction would be unsatisfactory. Perhaps the default strategy when establishing any new telemedicine system should be to consider prerecorded telemedicine first. Only if this appears unsatisfactory should one consider the use of realtime telemedicine as an alternative.

Types of realtime telemedicine

What kinds of information are transferred in a telemedicine interaction? Like prerecorded telemedicine, the interaction in a realtime telemedicine consultation can involve the transfer of various types of information:

- audio (i.e. the telephone);
- data, including text;
- still images;
- moving images (video).

Note that these categories are not mutually exclusive. Most realtime telemedicine will involve voice communication between the parties regardless

Table 4.2 Realtime telemedicine links

Category (and cost)	Type of information transmitted	Bandwidth
Low	Data, including text	2400 bit/s
Low	Audio (i.e. the telephone)	c35 kbit/s
Low/medium	Still images	28–128 kbit/s
Medium/high	Moving images (video)	128 kbit/s–150 Mbit/s

of what else it involves. Furthermore, the boundaries between the categories are not sharply defined. For example, the telephone network is often used in telemedicine to transmit data (with the aid of a modem), in addition to its conventional use for the transmission of audio.

The type of information to be transferred has implications for the connection required. Video is the most demanding and requires high-quality connections. For example, uncompressed video will require a very high bandwidth, up to 100 Mbit/s. On the other hand, physiological signals, such as a three-lead electrocardiographic (ECG) recording, can be transmitted over a low-speed data link at 2400 bit/s. See Table 4.2 for a summary.

Almost all current telemedicine involves the transmission of information relating to sight and sound. The other senses – smell, taste and touch – are not catered to. There has been some experimental work concerning the transmission of smell, but it will clearly be many years before suitable equipment is available for clinical trials. One area in which the transmission of smell might be useful is remote microbiology, since visual examination of culture plates is insufficient.[3]

Remote transmission of taste is theoretically possible, but there is no obvious demand for it in telemedicine (diabetes mellitus is diagnosed biochemically these days). On the other hand, transmission of touch would allow remote examination (e.g. palpation) to be performed without the aid of an amanuensis. Having to rely on someone else to perform the physical part of a remote examination is often said to be a restriction, although in practice it appears to cause remarkably little trouble. Haptic feedback devices, which convey the sensation of touch, are under development for remote surgery, so suitable technology may become available in due course.[4]

Realtime audio transfer

The use of the telephone is under-rated in telemedicine. One of the first questions when setting up a telemedicine system should be to ask what additional information would be conveyed by a picture and whether it is actually worth it.

It is often observed that there is a lack of evidence for cost-effectiveness in telemedicine. However, it is also true that certain forms of telemedicine, of which the use of the telephone is one, have never been formally evaluated. Yet it would be inconceivable to consider the practice of modern medicine without a telephone.

Telephone telemedicine includes the following.

Outpatient follow-up

Simple telephone follow-up of hospital outpatients has been shown to have advantages in some specialties. For example, rheumatology follow-up works well by telephone.[5] Orthopaedic assessments can also be done in the same way.[6] Such simple telemedicine techniques appear promising as a method of improving the efficiency of routine hospital-based clinics and deserve wider investigation.

Mental health

Psychiatry assessment and counselling are normally done face to face, but can also be carried out by telephone. Many of the standard test instruments have been validated for use by telephone.[7] Psychiatry assessment and treatment are possible by voice interaction with a computer.[8] Further details about telephone use in mental health are given by Wootton et al.[9]

Help lines

Starting in the 1990s, the UK National Health Service implemented a telephone help line for members of the public. The call centre provides 24 h telephone assistance in dealing with health-care emergencies and directs those needing assistance to the appropriate resource (e.g. general practitioner or hospital). The telephone service has been used enthusiastically by the public and the service has been extended to cover the whole of Britain. The majority of the calls to it occur outside normal working hours. One original aim of the service was to reduce pressure on hospital emergency departments, something which does not seem to have occurred.[10] There is also little evidence that it is cheaper than other methods of triage.[11] This is an example of a common situation in telemedicine, where an application provides a new service (i.e. out-of-hours access to a health professional), which is valued by the users, but which comes at an additional cost to society.

Support groups

Support groups can also 'meet' by telephone. For example, an audioconference network was established for rural breast cancer survivors in Canada. Self-help support sessions were held with up to 48 participants at 21 different sites. By sharing their experiences and providing mutual support, women in rural areas with breast cancer were able to overcome the isolation gap they experienced.[12] Similar mutual support was demonstrated in a randomized controlled trial among first-time, breast-feeding mothers.[13] The result was that significantly more mothers were breast-feeding at three months postpartum compared with those in the control group.

Realtime data transfer

Much telemonitoring is prerecorded since there is often no need for a realtime link. Realtime data transfer is indicated only if an immediate response is required.

Thus realtime transfer is used for teleconsultation in cardiology patients or other urgent cases. Data can be transferred over the ordinary public telephone network using a modem, or by fax. Data can also be transferred by mobile phone. Increasingly, the Internet is used for part of the communication pathway.

Modem

Data transmission by modem has been used for realtime blood pressure and realtime ECG monitoring of patients at home. ECG transmission has also been demonstrated from ambulances, using transmission via the mobile phone network. ECG monitoring from fixed locations has passed from the experimental stage to become a routine telecardiology service, with cardiac call centres set up to provide an immediate opinion from a cardiologist.[14]

Fax

Fax machines can be used to transfer paper records, such as ECG recordings. However, good-quality transmission of ECG traces is difficult without taking special precautions to digitize the recording appropriately. A fax machine was used to transmit surgical diagrams in a rural emergency to coach a rural general practitioner to perform a life-saving procedure.[15] Fax machines have also proven their value in telemedicine in the Antarctic.[16]

Mobile phone

The advantage of data transmission by fixed telephone line is that it can take place at rates of some 35 kbit/s and access to the telephone network is possible from almost anywhere in the world. Data transmission is also possible using a mobile phone, albeit at lower transmission rates and from more restricted areas. The key advantage is the mobility. Successful telemedicine has been carried out for cardiology, in which an ECG was transmitted to a mobile phone with a built-in display.[17] Long-term peak flow monitoring has been performed in 91 asthmatic patients using mobile phones to transmit the data to a central server for an average duration of 203 days.[18]

Realtime still image transfer

The most mature application in telemedicine generally is teleradiology. In the vast majority of cases this involves the transfer of still images in prerecorded mode. There are circumstances in which this is also done in realtime, usually as part of a realtime teleconsultation. However, the most common application in which still images are transferred in realtime is telepathology.

Telepathology

Telepathology remains an active area of research. Certain forms of telepathology are well suited to prerecorded telemedicine (see Chapter 3). However, when an immediate diagnosis is required, for example during a surgical operation, realtime

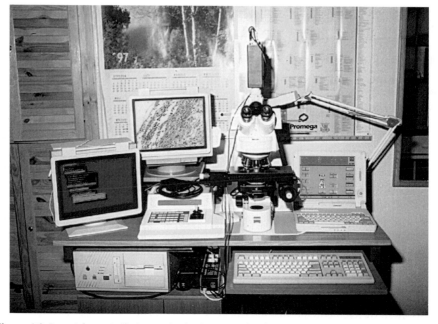

Figure 4.1 Remotely controlled motorized microscope for the transmission of colour video pictures (Photo credit: K Kayser)

telepathology must be used. One of the earliest realtime telepathology services began in Norway in 1990. The frozen-section service was provided from the University Hospital in Tromsø to peripheral hospitals in northern Norway.[19] Similar services are now offered from Trondheim, using remotely controlled microscopes with a network connection of sufficient bandwidth to allow the transmission of medium-quality colour video pictures. In practice, most diagnoses can be made on the basis of the realtime video pictures (Figure 4.1), without the need to transmit high-resolution still pictures as well.

Teleradiology

Realtime teleconsultation between physicians in different hospitals has been demonstrated using videoconferencing for face-to-face interaction, combined with the simultaneous transfer of still images in a parallel data channel. This allows a radiologist to discuss a case with the referring doctor while both examine the same images. Such techniques, while probably providing an improved standard of care, remain too expensive for routine use.

Mobile phone links, which have the advantage of wireless connection, have been used to transfer radiology images to notebook computers for reporting by the radiologists on duty out of hours. In a study of 30 emergency head computerized tomography studies, there were no major discrepancies in 82 out of 90 interpretations (91%), suggesting that portable radiology workstations may permit radiologists to provide rapid consultations from anywhere within the mobile phone coverage area.[20]

Accident and emergency telemedicine

Attempts to improve communication between emergency ambulances transporting patients and the staff at the receiving hospital have centred on the use of mobile phone links to transmit data such as ECG signals. This allows, for example, prehospital thrombolysis to be started by paramedical staff before arrival at hospital, thus reducing call-to-needle times.[21] Still images have also been sent from ambulances and transmission rates of about 15 pictures/min are possible.[22] Widespread use of image transmission will probably depend on better telecommunications.

Once the patient has arrived at hospital, mobile phones with built-in cameras can be useful in obtaining a second opinion. There have been encouraging trials in wound care and in burns.[23,24] In one trial of teleconsultation in injuries to fingers, the mean time between taking photographs to their reception was 3–4 min.

Realtime video transfer

Realtime telemedicine involving video transmission has been used successfully in a number of specialties.

Telepsychiatry

Telepsychiatry is arguably the most successful realtime telemedicine application. It is not easily done in prerecorded mode, although psychotherapy by email has been reported. Realtime telepsychiatry, i.e. videoconferencing, is one of the few telemedicine applications for which there is some formal evidence of its efficacy and effectiveness.[25] Much of the work in Australia was originally done at low bandwidths (128 kbit/s) and much of the work in the US began at much higher bandwidths (1.54 Mbit/s). Current preference in both countries seems to be for telepsychiatry at a bandwidth of about 384 kbit/s. Further details about the use of realtime video in psychiatry are given by Wootton et al.[9]

Tele-ENT

Much of the published experience in ENT consultation by telemedicine concerns realtime interaction using video endoscopy.[26] It is clear that tele-ENT can be an effective method of consultation between a primary care practitioner and a specialist (Figure 4.2). Unnecessary referrals can be avoided and there may be early detection of serious pathology. Although the telemedicine equipment is likely to be relatively expensive, a high enough patient workload can achieve savings in comparison with patients' travel to a specialist centre.[2]

It is also possible to carry out ENT consultation on the basis of prerecorded interaction, e.g. using still images or short video clips. There are not yet many

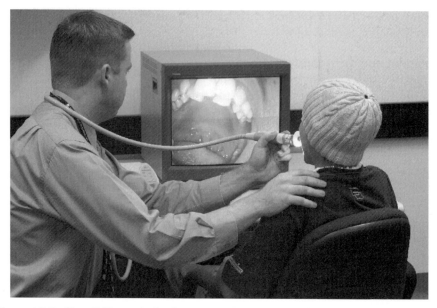

Figure 4.2 Realtime ENT consultation between a primary care practitioner and a specialist (Photo credit: R Wootton)

studies that compare the two methods. In one study of 45 patients,[27] there were no significant differences between the realtime telemedicine diagnosis and the conventional face-to-face diagnosis. However, only in 62% of the prerecorded cases were the video clips judged to provide sufficient information for a diagnosis. As is the case with teledermatology, there are likely to be situations in which realtime tele-ENT is superior and also situations in which prerecorded tele-ENT is superior.

Accident and emergency telemedicine

In contrast to some specialties (e.g. teledermatology), accident and emergency (A&E) telemedicine must be realtime, because the delays in prerecorded mode are unacceptable. There is substantial experience of realtime teleconsultation in the US.[28] Brennan *et al.*[29] carried out a randomized controlled trial of A&E telemedicine and found it to be satisfactory for a range of non-life-threatening conditions. The technique offers the possibility of improving support for small-hospital emergency departments, especially out of normal working hours.

In the UK, telemedicine has been very successful as a decision-support aid for nurse practitioners running minor injury services in the absence of on-the-spot medical cover (Figure 4.3). Regional minor injuries networks are beginning to evolve, based on main A&E departments at tertiary hospitals.[30]

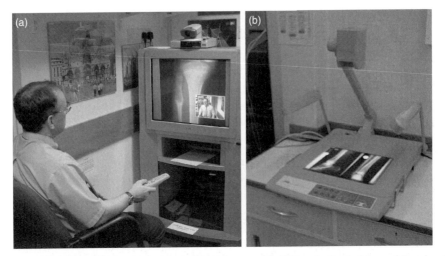

Figure 4.3 Realtime telemedicine for decision support: (a) A&E consultant giving advice about fracture management; (b) X-ray transmission using a document camera (Photo credit: J Ferguson)

Teledermatology

Teledermatology can be practised by prerecorded techniques, for example involving the capture of still images using a digital camera and their transmission to a specialist using email. Teledermatology can also be done in realtime and there is as yet no general agreement about which method is best. It may in fact turn out to be the case that each technique has particular advantages under certain circumstances, and that neither is to be preferred over the other.[31]

Realtime teledermatology can be done using expensive equipment: high-resolution, high-magnification videocameras ('dermascopes') and high-bandwidth transmission; or it can be done using relatively low-cost videocameras and narrowband ISDN connections.[32] Again, there is no general agreement about which is preferable, and this may turn out to be a sterile area for debate. What is striking about the field of teledermatology as a whole – both prerecorded and realtime – is how little quantitative information exists about the diagnostic accuracy and the quality of management advice that can be delivered. It is also true, *en passant*, that relatively little is known about these factors in conventional, face-to-face dermatology.

Teleneurology

Transmission of electroencephalography (EEG) data was first done in Canada using the telephone network. Eight-channel recordings were transmitted to the regional centre for interpretation. Realtime transmission of 32-channel EEG data with simultaneous videoconferencing has been used in Finland for patients with a range of neurological problems. A high-bandwidth, fibre-optic link was required. More recently, the use of lower-cost videolinks has been shown to be satisfactory for remote examination of acute neurology patients. Some problems that can be solved by realtime teleneurology include:

(1) patients admitted to hospital with acute neurological symptoms rarely seeing a neurologist;
(2) delayed treatment for acute stroke;
(3) non-optimum management of epilepsy;
(4) unproductive travel time for neurologists;
(5) long waiting times to see a neurologist.

Realtime teleneurology is also useful in the management of stroke. For further details about the use of realtime video in neurology see Wootton and Patterson.[33]

Teleoncology

Most of the experience with practising oncology by telemedicine has been obtained in Kansas, where it has been used very successfully for direct patient care.[34] Realtime telemedicine has also been used for radiotherapy planning and for case conferencing in multidisciplinary oncology meetings with a tertiary referral centre. In Kansas, tele-oncology has considerable advantages in allowing patients to be treated locally and reducing travel for doctors who would otherwise conduct outreach clinics in peripheral hospitals. Formal evidence for cost-effectiveness remains to be obtained, but preliminary indications are encouraging.

Teledialysis

Telemedicine has been used successfully to support renal dialysis patients in satellite hospitals. In South Australia, the regional dialysis unit in Adelaide has carried out several thousand consultations using low-bandwidth videolinks (128 kbit/s).[35] In Texas, higher-quality videolinks have been used, also very successfully.[36] Experiments are taking place to extend the support of hospital renal departments to patients being dialysed at home. As in other telecare applications, videoconferencing to the home is critically dependent on the availability of appropriate bandwidth.

Decision support for remote practitioners

Realtime telemedicine is particularly valuable as a decision support aid for practitioners in remote locations such as the Antarctic.[16] However, telemedicine may also be useful in urban conurbations. Its use for minor injuries units has been mentioned above. The success of telemedicine services for school nurses in the US is noteworthy.[37] Telemedicine has also been used to provide access to psychiatry services from inner city, deprived areas and as a means of supporting intensive-care units in smaller hospitals by sharing specialized staff between them.

Intermediate between truly isolated regions, such as the Antarctic, and large metropolitan areas, where travel can be slow, are the innumerable relatively small hospitals that serve local communities in regional and rural areas. Telemedicine can be used to good effect to support the practice of medicine in such hospitals, using specialist expertise located in tertiary hospitals in large cities. This seems to work especially well in many areas of paediatrics (see Wootton and Batch[38] for further details of telepaediatrics), including the transmission of live ultrasound scans to cardiologists or fetal medicine specialists.

Other

For similar reasons – providing access to medical services where there is no alternative – telemedicine has been used for decades at sea. Most of the major maritime nations established radio medical services for merchant ships in the early part of the 20th century. By the 1990s, for example, the Italian radio medical service had dealt with over 40,000 patients, mainly on ships, and more recently had provided assistance in the case of airline passengers becoming ill during a flight (about 1% of the workload).[39]

Telemedicine for passenger aircraft is a particularly interesting area in view of the high costs of diverting long-haul aircraft if a medical emergency occurs. The major airlines experience significant numbers of such diversions and medical advice is normally provided from the ground via a radio link to the duty doctor.[40] Transmission of vital signs in flight may allow better decision making about whether a diversion is appropriate.

Tele-education

Distance education in medicine often involves videoconferencing between teacher and students. Removing the need for the participants to travel has major advantages in rural areas, and tele-education has been used successfully by doctors, nurses and allied health staff in rural areas. Interactive distance teaching has also been used for undergraduate medical education. Note that huge amounts of education are now done in non-realtime using the Web; this is obviously a cheaper technique, although it does not have the advantage of live interaction with the teacher. For a recent review of telemedicine and continuing medical education, see Rafiq and Merrell.[41]

Satellite broadcasting is a method of delivering medical education. If the broadcast was unidirectional then there would be few advantages over the transmission of the same material on prerecorded videocassettes, so satellite education in medicine usually contains an interactive component. Unfortunately, the cost of satellite transmission is very high, and several pioneering educational programmes have ultimately proved to be unsustainable. Video transmission via terrestrial networks seems to be a more affordable technique.

Choosing a system

Yellowlees has identified seven factors which appear to be critical in the successful development of telemedicine programmes (see Chapter 7). At the earlier stage of establishing telemedicine systems, there are seven key questions which should be asked:

(1) What is the *clinical problem* to be solved? This is the crux of the matter.
(2) What is the *background*? For example:
  • If a conventional face-to-face referral is easy, why bother with distance medicine?
  • Will the participants accept telemedicine? Patients are usually enthusiastic about telemedicine, but medical staff cannot be assumed to be so. It is likely to be important to identify clearly the benefits to the practitioners involved.
  • What would be the advantages of telemedicine? For example, what would be the financial savings and who would receive them?
(3) What *organizational changes* will be required to take advantage of telemedicine? Also, what organizational changes can be expected (e.g. altered referral patterns) and will they be accepted by those involved?
(4) What is the right telemedicine *technique* to be used: realtime or prerecorded? This should not be viewed as an exclusive choice. In some circumstances, a hybrid model, combining both realtime and prerecorded, may be advantageous
(5) Who will be responsible for *training and support*? It is particularly important to understand that both of these will be continuing requirements.
(6) What is the minimum *quality* of equipment required? For example:
  • Is video required, or will audio alone suffice?
  • If video is required, will 10–15 frames/s suffice or must it be 25–30?
(7) What *technology* is required? Choice of equipment should be left until all the foregoing matters have been resolved. Furthermore, a minimalist approach should be adopted in specifying the equipment required. One of the striking features of failed or failing telemedicine projects is the number of expensive peripherals which have been purchased but never used, such as dermascopes and electronic stethoscopes.

Conclusion

Telemedicine in general, and realtime telemedicine in particular, can work very well given the right circumstance. Since prerecorded telemedicine is both cheaper and more convenient than realtime, the use of the latter should not be contemplated unless prerecorded telemedicine will not meet the clinical objectives.

Some realtime telemedicine applications have been taken up with enthusiasm, even if formal evidence of cost-effectiveness may be lacking. Teleradiology and telepsychiatry are two examples where widespread adoption is beginning to occur. Other forms of realtime telemedicine represent 'niche' applications. That is, they appear to be both successful and sustainable in the centres where they were pioneered, but have not been adopted elsewhere. Teledialysis and teleoncology are examples of this type. The patchy diffusion of telemedicine is something that is not yet well understood.

References

1   Grigsby B. *2004 TRC Report on US Telemedicine Activity*. Kingston, NJ: Civic Research Institute, 2004
2   Bergmo TS. An economic analysis of teleconsultation in otorhinolaryngology. *J Telemed Telecare* 1997;**3**:194–9
3   Akselsen S, Hartviksen G, Vorland L. Remote interpretation of microbiology specimens based on transmitted still images. *J Telemed Telecare* 1995;**1**:229–33
4   Stalfors J, Kling-Petersen T, Rydmark M, Westin T. Haptic palpation of head and neck cancer patients – implication for education and telemedicine. *Stud Health Technol Inform* 2001;**81**:471–4
5   Pal B. Tele-rheumatology: telephone follow up and cyberclinic. *Comput Methods Programs Biomed* 2001;**64**:189–95
6   Sharma S, Shah R, Draviraj KP, Bhamra MS. Use of telephone interviews to follow up patients after total hip replacement. *J Telemed Telecare* 2005;**11**:211–4
7   Rohde P, Lewinsohn PM, Seeley JR. Comparability of telephone and face-to-face interviews in assessing axis I and II disorders. *Am J Psychiatry* 1997;**154**:1593–8
8   Bachofen M, Nakagawa A, Marks IM, *et al*. Home self-assessment and self-treatment of obsessive–compulsive disorder using a manual and a computer-conducted telephone interview: replication of a UK–US study. *J Clin Psychiatry* 1999;**60**:545–9
9   Wootton R, Yellowlees P, McLaren P, eds. *Telepsychiatry and e-Mental Health*. London: Royal Society of Medicine Press, 2003
10 Munro J, Nicholl J, O'Cathain A, Knowles E. Impact of NHS direct on demand for immediate care: observational study. *BMJ* 2000;**321**:150–3
11 Richards DA, Godfrey L, Tawfik J, *et al*. NHS Direct versus general practice based triage for same day appointments in primary care: cluster randomised controlled trial. *BMJ* 2004;**329**:774
12 Curran VR, Church JG. A study of rural women's satisfaction with a breast cancer self-help network. *J Telemed Telecare* 1999;**5**:47–54
13 Dennis CL, Hodnett E, Gallop R, Chalmers B. The effect of peer support on breast-feeding duration among primiparous women: a randomized controlled trial. *CMAJ* 2002;**166**:21–8
14 Scalvini S, Zanelli E, Conti C, *et al*. Assessment of prehospital chest pain using telecardiology. *J Telemed Telecare* 2002;**8**:231–236
15 Rottger J, Irving AM, Broere J, Tranmer B. Use of telecommunications in a rural emergency. Brain surgery by fax. *J Telemed Telecare* 1997;**3**:59–60
16 Hyer RN. Telemedical experiences at an Antarctic station. *J Telemed Telecare* 1999;**5** (Suppl. 1):87–9
17 Freedman SB. Direct transmission of electrocardiograms to a mobile phone for management of a patient with acute myocardial infarction. *J Telemed Telecare* 1999;**5**:67–9
18 Ryan D, Cobern W, Wheeler J, Price D, Tarassenko L. Mobile phone technology in the management of asthma. *J Telemed Telecare* 2005;**11** (Suppl. 1):43–6
19 Nordrum I, Engum B, Rinde E, *et al*. Remote frozen section service: a telepathology project in northern Norway. *Hum Pathol* 1991;**22**:514–8
20 Pagani L, Jyrkinen L, Niinimaki J, *et al*. A portable diagnostic workstation based on a Webpad: implementation and evaluation. *J Telemed Telecare* 2003;**9**:225–9
21 Pedley DK, Beedie S, Ferguson J. Mobile telemetry for pre-hospital thrombolysis: problems and solutions. *J Telemed Telecare* 2005;**11** (Suppl. 1):78–80
22 Curry GR, Harrop N. The Lancashire telemedicine ambulance. *J Telemed Telecare* 1998;**4**:231–8
23 Braun RP, Vecchietti JL, Thomas L, *et al*. Telemedical wound care using a new generation of mobile telephones: a feasibility study. *Arch Dermatol* 2005;**141**:254–8
24 Hsieh CH, Tsai HH, Yin JW, Chen CY, Yang JC, Jeng SF. Teleconsultation with the mobile camera-phone in digital soft-tissue injury: a feasibility study. *Plast Reconstr Surg* 2004;**114**:1776–82
25 Hailey D, Roine R, Ohinmaa A. Systematic review of evidence for the benefits of telemedicine. *J Telemed Telecare* 2002;**8** (Suppl. 1):1–30
26 Haegen TW, Cupp CC, Hunsaker DH. Teleotolaryngology: a retrospective review at a military tertiary treatment facility. *Otolaryngol Head Neck Surg* 2004;**130**:511–8

27   Stern J, Heneghan C, Sclafani AP, Ginsburg J, Sabini P, Dolitsky JN. Telemedicine applications in otolaryngology. *J Telemed Telecare* 1998;**4** (Suppl. 1):74–5

28   Lambrecht CJ. Telemedicine in trauma care: description of 100 trauma teleconsults. *Telemed J* 1997;**3**:265–8

29   Brennan JA, Kealy JA, Gerardi LH, *et al.* Telemedicine in the emergency department: a randomized controlled trial. *J Telemed Telecare* 1999;**5**:18–22

30   Ferguson J, Rowlands A, Palombo A, Pedley D, Fraser S, Simpson S. Minor injuries telemedicine. *J Telemed Telecare* 2003;**9** (Suppl. 1):14–16

31   Wootton R, Oakley AMM, eds. *Teledermatology.* London: Royal Society of Medicine Press, 2002

32   Wootton R, Bloomer SE, Corbett R, *et al.* Multicentre randomised control trial comparing real time teledermatology with conventional outpatient dermatological care: societal cost-benefit analysis. *BMJ* 2000;**320**:1252–6

33   Wootton R, Patterson V. *Teleneurology.* London: Royal Society of Medicine Press, 2005

34   Doolittle GC. Telemedicine in Kansas: the successes and the challenges. *J Telemed Telecare* 2001;**7** (Suppl. 2):43–6

35   Mitchell JG, Disney AP. Clinical applications of renal telemedicine. *J Telemed Telecare* 1997;**3**:158–162

36   Moncrief JW. Telemedicine in the care of the end-stage renal disease patient. *Adv Ren Replace Ther* 1998;**5**:286–91

37   Young TL, Ireson C. Effectiveness of school-based telehealth care in urban and rural elementary schools. *Pediatrics* 2003;**112**:1088–94

38   Wootton R, Batch J, eds. *Telepediatrics: Telemedicine and Child Health.* London: Royal Society of Medicine Press, 2004

39   Amenta F, Dauri A, Rizzo N. Organization and activities of the International Radio Medical Centre (CIRM). *J Telemed Telecare* 1996;**2**:125–31

40   Bagshaw M. Telemedicine in British Airways. *J Telemed Telecare* 1996;**2** (Suppl. 1):36–8

41   Rafiq A, Merrell RC. Telemedicine for access to quality care on medical practice and continuing medical education in a global arena. *J Contin Educ Health Prof* 2005;**25**:34–42

Further information

1   Maheu M, Whitten P, Allen A. *E-Health, Telehealth, and Telemedicine: A Guide to Startup and Success.* San Francisco: Jossey-Bass, 2001

2   Dodd AZ. *Essential Guide to Telecommunications.* NJ: Prentice-Hall, 2000

3   Wootton R, Batch J, eds. *Telepediatrics: Telemedicine and Child Health.* London: Royal Society of Medicine Press, 2004

▶5

Tele-education

Vernon R Curran

Introduction

Health professionals have a commitment to continued study and lifelong learning. As a result, health-care professionals employ many methods to stay abreast of new information and to meet their continuing education needs. Formal and informal activities can include attending rounds, reading books and journals, discussing papers with peers, attending conferences, workshops and lectures, and using video and audiotape devices. However, a critical issue and challenge for health-care professionals in rural areas is the difficulty they encounter in receiving and participating in continuing education.

Tele-education, defined as the application of information and communication technologies (ICTs) in the delivery of distance learning, has been used for many years to deliver continuing education programmes to rural health-care professionals. Tele-education delivery modes are distinguished according to the technologies and medium used. The main categories of tele-education delivery modes are audio, video and computer. In the 1990s, there were significant advances in information and communication technology. These developments enabled a new generation of technologies for facilitating tele-education.

Audio technologies

Audio technologies involve the transmission of the spoken word (voice) between learners and instructors. There are two main types: synchronous or asynchronous. The synchronous technologies enable realtime communication between two or more health-care professionals. Audioconferencing and short-wave radio are examples of the synchronous audio-mediated technologies which have been reported in the continuing education literature. The main difference between the two is that audioconferencing (i.e. by telephone) allows 'many-to-many' interactive communication, while radio only allows 'one-to-many'.

Asynchronous audio technologies transmit verbal information for subsequent playback and review. The audiotape or audiocassette is an example of an asynchronous technology which has been used for providing distance learning to health professionals.

Audioconferencing

Audioconferencing (Figure 5.1) has been used for continuing education for health professionals since the 1960s.[1] Its use for tele-education has been reported in several studies from the US and Canada.[2-5] In one study, audioconferencing was used internationally, between the Emergency Hospital of Yerevan, Armenia, and the Boston University School of Medicine to provide formal opportunities for continuing medical education (CME) for physicians in Armenia.[6]

An audioconferencing system may incorporate telephones that have loudspeakers and microphones embedded in the base component of a handset. Such equipment allows large-scale audioconferences to be established with groups of participants at multiple sites. Thus, several participants can participate in a conference discussion.

Audio bridges, or linking devices, are used to link telephones or conferencing sites together so the parties at all locations can hear and talk to each other. Access to a telecommunications bridge is usually through a telecommunications service provider or sometimes through educational institutions that use audio-conferencing to support distance-learning programmes.

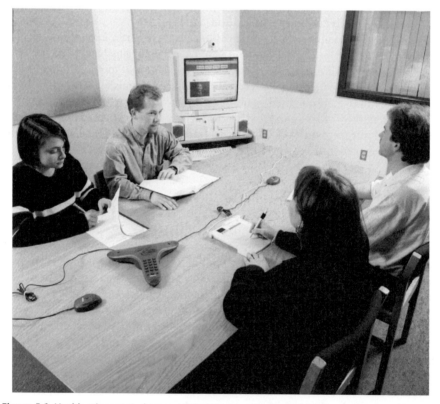

Figure 5.1 Health sciences students participating in an audioconference supplemented by Web-enabled conferencing software

The department of Continuing Medical Education at the University of Wisconsin, Madison, began to use audioconferencing for continuing education delivery in 1965.[1] Audioconferencing facilities were installed in 18 hospitals across the state with the furthest sites up to 550 km from Madison. In the mid-1970s the network had expanded to over 170 different locations throughout the state, and between 1966 and 1976 more than 28,000 nurses in Wisconsin had participated in continuing education programmes over the system.[7] Today, the Educational Telephone Network (ETN) of the state of Wisconsin is a closed-access telephone network which links university health science departments and resources in the state's capital of Madison with learners around the state. The University of Wisconsin Extension Division and the Departments of Continuing Medical Education, Nursing and Pharmacy collaborate to offer hundreds of hours annually of educational programmes to the state's hospitals.

In Newfoundland and Labrador, a similar audioconferencing network was developed during the late 1960s to provide CME to the many rural physicians practising in isolated locations along the province's coastline. The CME department at the Faculty of Medicine organized weekly, hour-long audio-conference sessions.[3] The audioconference system operated like a modified party line with groups of physicians in different hospitals using microphone and speaker equipment instead of telephones.

Short-wave radio

Use of radio to augment continuing education activities began in 1955 when the Albany Medical College began broadcasting programmes to physicians and pharmacists in the north-east of the US.[8] Using a frequency modulation (FM) radio station, staff at the Medical College delivered hour-long presentations to participants in several New England states. The presenters could also hear questions from participants via a special telephone connection and provide live answers. Other universities followed suit and similar radio programmes were developed by various colleges of medicine, mainly in the US.

Radio has also been used to deliver continuing education programmes in Australia and Europe. In Australia, a radio network covering most of the isolated parts of the continent has enabled the majority of remote nurses to access continuing education material.[9] In Finland, the Finnish Centre of Continuing Pharmaceutical Education, together with the Finnish Broadcasting Company and the University of Kuopio, arranged a radio series in 1990 for pharmacists and pharmacist assistants.[10] A survey indicated that 57% of the respondents had listened to some of the programmes. The most common barrier to listening to the transmission was an unsuitable broadcast time. A large number of the respondents to the survey felt that the programmes were useful to them, but the lack of opportunity for interaction with instructors and other participants was reported as the main problem with instruction by radio.

Video technologies

Video for distance learning, like audio, can be used in either synchronous or asynchronous fashion. Videoconferencing or interactive television technologies are considered synchronous because there is the opportunity for live visual and verbal interaction between instructors and learners.[11] Asynchronous instructional video tools include slow-scan video, interactive videodiscs and videotapes.

Videoconferencing

Videoconferencing systems have experienced significant growth in recent years because of increased digital transmission options at reduced costs, improvements in video compression technologies and improvements in the systems with an associated decrease in their cost. Videoconferencing technology is often installed in hospitals for health-care delivery purposes (i.e. for telehealth or telemedicine). The main interest in videoconferencing for educational purposes is because of

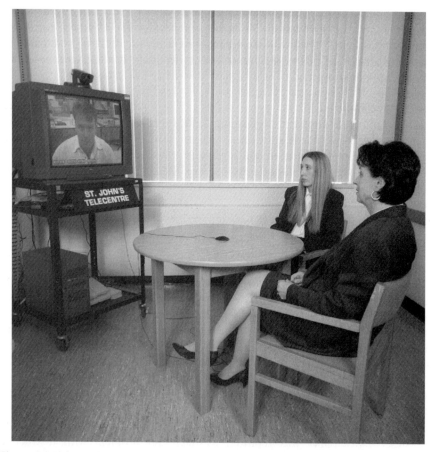

Figure 5.2 Videoconferencing using a roll-about conferencing system

the interactive communication which it permits. This enables instructors to receive immediate feedback from participants, allowing them to adjust their presentations accordingly[12] (Figure 5.2). Videoconferences can be of two types: point-to-point or multipoint. In point-to-point conferences, the communication and interaction occur only between two sites. Multipoint videoconferencing involves more than two sites and is accomplished by using a 'bridge' which links the various locations.

Videoconferencing is typically delivered using satellite, fibre-optic cable or digital connections (e.g. ISDN lines). Satellite transmission involves sending the signal from a videoconferencing studio to an orbiting telecommunications satellite from where the signal is beamed to reception sites, e.g. at universities or hospitals.[13] This method can be very expensive. Fibre-optic cable is often cheaper, but is possible only where the necessary infrastructure is available in the required locations. In rural and remote areas where fibre-optic cables are not available, videoconferencing can be accomplished over digital lines using a piece of computer equipment called a codec.

The codec compresses the information contained in a video transmission, and its accompanying audio signal, into a smaller bandwidth (see Chapter 2). The resultant data are transmitted to the remote end of the videoconferencing link, where the digital signals are then decoded into analogue video and audio.[12] The equipment required for videoconferencing does not need to be massive or expensive. Roll-about units are available that can turn any conference room into a videoconference facility quickly and easily. At the higher end of the price scale are more elaborate, more permanent types of conference installations with built-in permanent videoconferencing centres that can be situated where the demand justifies them (see Chapter 2).

Broadcast and closed-circuit television

There are three methods for transmitting television pictures: (1) open-circuit (also known as broadcast) systems; (2) open-circuit, but scrambled, image systems; and (3) closed-circuit systems.[14] Broadcast television allows for one-way video and audio transmissions to multiple receiving sites. One of the first groups in the field of medical education television was the Medical Television Network (MTN) operated by the University of California Extension, Los Angeles (UCLA). MTN began with weekly broadcasts of continuing education programmes to physicians and nurses in 72 hospitals in southern California using a scrambled (encoded) broadcast system.

In Canada, broadcast television began in the late 1960s. The Faculty of Medicine at the University of Western Ontario used broadcast television for continuing education programmes for approximately 2200 doctors in south-western Ontario.[15] It was estimated that 900–1000 viewers watched at least one of the broadcasts and half of these could have been regarded as regular viewers.

The Intercollegiate Center for Nursing Education (ICNE) based in Spokane, Washington, has been using broadcast and cable television to deliver continuing education courses since 1980.[16] The participants in these programmes received printed materials to supplement the transmissions, and were able to request continuing education credit by completing an end-of-unit examination. Programmes were originally broadcast via several cable channels on the state public broadcasting system (PBS). These programmes were live productions, so participants in the workplace could interact with faculty members in the classroom by a telephone in a one-way video, two-way audio loop.

Closed-circuit television systems utilize a localized (closed) broadcast network for transmitting one-way audio and video information, and are usually located within a given institution or region. The Division of Continuing Education at the Louisiana State University (LSU) School of Medicine used closed-circuit television to offer a monthly two-hour CME television programme to over 20 hospitals via the statewide Louisiana Hospital Television Network.[17] The network had a two-way talk-back system, which allowed viewers to comment and ask questions on air. The Emory Medical Television Network provided medical institutions in the Atlanta area with educational programmes through its Instructional Television Fixed Services (ITFS). ITFS was a closed-circuit, two-way TV system that allowed an audience in diverse remote locations to view, via TV, lectures and intricate demonstrations. The network was self-supporting and broadcasts included three hours of live, full-colour programming.

Satellite TV

Television programmes can be transmitted via a satellite and received by a dish, rather than by a rooftop aerial or a cable network.[18] Many hospitals have subscribed to satellite networks to provide programming to meet the educational needs of health-care professionals. An instructional session (live or recorded) can be transmitted from a studio through an earth station to a satellite. The satellite carries transponders, which re-transmit the coded signals to receivers within the satellite footprint (that is, the transmission area covered by the satellite). A satellite dish, usually on the roof of the hospital, receives the signal, which is then decoded and viewed on television monitors.

In Canada, the use of satellites dates back to the 1970s, when the technology was used in the delivery of CME to physicians in rural and remote regions.[19] Several projects in education and telehealth were piloted using the Hermes satellite. A two-way audio and video link between the Moose Factory hospital and the University Hospital in London, Ontario, enabled both continuing education and telehealth consultations.

Videotapes

Videotapes have played an important role in tele-education over the years. With the widespread availability of videocassette players (VCRs), videotapes have become a very convenient and cost-effective way of disseminating instructional materials to rural and remote health-care professionals. Most individuals have access to a VCR, whether in their home or their workplace, and videotapes are relatively inexpensive to distribute. The videotape, and video in general, is a good medium for teaching interpersonal skills and for teaching procedures, since it can show the sequence and actions involved. In one recent example, videotapes were used to provide CME on interpersonal violence to physicians and other personnel (e.g. nurses, social workers) at 24 sites associated with four academic medical centres.[20] Videotapes were found to be an efficient way of providing training in these multiple locations and effective in improving knowledge and attitudes about child, elder, sexual and domestic violence. The videotape programme was also rated highly by clinicians from the different fields.

Computer-mediated learning technologies

The terminology which is used to refer to computer-mediated learning varies. Computer-assisted learning (CAL) or instruction (CAI) can be defined as any learning that is mediated by a computer and which requires no direct interaction between the user and a human instructor in order to run. CAL is becoming an increasingly common method of enhancing nursing and medical education due to its ability to simulate clinical conditions and its versatility in providing a self-directed educational resource with around-the-clock access. Computer applications in distance learning have also been referred to as computer-managed instruction (CMI), computer-based training (CBT) and in recent times online, Web-based or e-learning. Examples of present-day computer-mediated technologies in tele-education include: the Internet and World Wide Web, email, synchronous and asynchronous computer-mediated communication applications, and interactive multimedia applications on CD-ROM.

Internet and the World Wide Web
The growth of the Internet and the World Wide Web has created new opportunities for tele-education. The role of the Internet as a source of information for physicians has grown rapidly since the inception of the Web. One factor which has contributed to this growth is the increasing and complex information needs of physicians. The tremendous growth in medical knowledge is a challenge for physicians, who are expected to maintain their knowledge on the most recent advances in medicine. Kripalani et al.[21] have suggested that the Internet is a valuable source of information which can be used to assist physicians in addressing patient questions. In one recent study, 2200 primary-care physicians were surveyed about medical information-seeking behaviours and use of the Internet.[22] Nearly all physicians reported access to the Internet, knew how to use it and used it for locating medical information. The most common reason for seeking information was to solve a particular patient problem. Casebeer et al.[22] found that the main importance of the Internet to physicians was in the area of professional development and information seeking to provide better care. The ability to scan a wide range of information makes the Internet a unique support

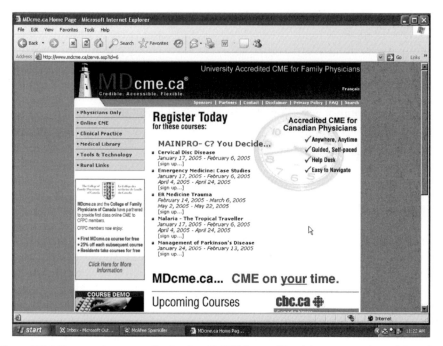

Figure 5.3 MDcme.ca is an accredited online CME Web portal involving a consortium of Canadian university CME departments (http://www.mdcme.ca)

tool for a self-directed curriculum. It is possible for physicians to develop and manage their own self-directed curriculum by drawing on different kinds of resources at different times through the Internet.

The Internet offers a new dimension for facilitating CME for physician audiences.[23] The Web is an ideal medium for delivering CME because information is universally available, easily updated and quickly obtained, and CME can easily be delivered to the site of clinical activity. Web-based CME is also advantageous because it allows the user to select the content, pace and place of learning. It allows physicians to obtain CME from regional, national and international experts without the need to travel (Figure 5.3). The main benefits of Web-based CME include easy access, low cost, multimedia format and an ability to create interactive clinical cases. The Web also enables the presentation of ideas in ways that would be impossible in printed text, using multimedia components such as sound and movies.

As Internet usage has grown, there has been a significant increase in the number of Web-based CME providers and the number of CME Websites.[24] In 2000, 96 CME sites were available and by 2001 this number had increased to 200. Web-based CME programmes delivered through a variety of formats and provided by an array of organizations and institutions are available online. CME credit may be received by reading, viewing or listening to online learning materials or media, and in some instances by completing an interactive quiz.

The design of these Web-based CME programmes varies, as does the process through which learning is facilitated. High-quality online professional learning opportunities may provide physicians with new options for accessing the best educational programmes that medicine has to offer.[25] There may also be new opportunities to interact with expert faculty members, integrate newly published or peer-reviewed scientific information and clinical developments, and improve the process of taking courses and tracking credits.

Current state of tele-education

Several studies have examined the use of tele-education technologies among North American health professional education providers. Members of the American Association of Colleges of Nursing were surveyed to determine the state of the art in distance-learning technology use.[26] The results indicated an increase in course offerings through distance-learning technologies. A Web-based survey of North American CME providers and the distance-learning technologies they employed has also been carried out.[27] The results suggest that the majority of providers had not developed distance education programmes.

A recent survey of the current state of tele-education among Canadian providers of continuing health-professional education produced some interesting findings.[28] The survey population included academic institutions (schools of medicine, nursing and pharmacy), national/provincial health-professional associations, the pharmaceutical industry and hospital/health-care authority organizations. Physicians and nurses comprise the largest health professional groups in the country, and they also comprise the largest groups in rural and remote regions of Canada. The survey results suggest that Canadian schools of medicine and nursing report the greatest level of experience in tele-education and are responsible for a significant proportion of the distance-learning programming which is provided to health professionals.

Factors related to financial gain do not appear to have a significant influence on an academic continuing education provider's decision to provide distance learning. Such providers indicated that they were more likely to provide tele-education as a means for addressing the needs of rural and remote health professionals, to increase opportunities for flexible continuing education access and to fulfil an organization's mission. Hospital and health-care management boards favour tele-education as a more cost-effective means of addressing the mandatory continuing education needs of health professionals.

The survey findings also indicated that Internet-based technologies (e.g. email and the World Wide Web) and videoconferencing were the most common tele-education technologies being used. Existing learning technology resources and expertise (human, technical and infrastructure) within an organization or institution appeared to be important factors which influenced the likelihood that a provider offers tele-education programming.

CME in the future

Rural health-care professionals need timely, appropriate and evidence-based learning resources for continuous knowledge and skill development so that they can provide a competent level of health-care service. A common deterrent to practice in rural and remote areas is lack of access to professional development. The delivery of tele-education programmes via information and communications technologies enables the dissemination of new developments, provides training opportunities for hospital staff and employees, and enhances educational experiences for primary care practitioners through consultations with specialists and virtual attendance at academic grand rounds. The use of such techniques has the potential to alleviate some of the isolation felt by rural health-care professionals, and it reduces the costs, travel time and staff absences associated with distant continuing education programming.[29]

Tele-education technologies have an important role to play in addressing the professional isolation which is experienced by rural and remote health-care professionals.

References

1   Meyer TC. Teleconferencing as a medium for continuing education of health professionals. *Mobius* 1983;**3**:73–9
2   McDowell CA, Challis EB, Lockyer JM, White L, Adams K, Parboosingh IJ. Teleconferencing CME programs to rural physicians: the University of Calgary teleconference program. *Can Fam Physician* 1987;**33**:1705–8
3   House AM, Roberts JM, Canning EM. Telemedicine provides new dimensions in CME in Newfoundland and Labrador. *Can Med Assoc J* 1981;**124**:801–2
4   Parker LA, Baird MA. Continuing education by telephone: a party line for professionals. *Hospitals* 1977;**51**:105–6, 108, 110–12
5   Gellman EF, Franke TC. Experience with four years of CME teleconferencing at St Louis Children's Hospital, Washington University School of Medicine. *J Contin Educ Health Prof* 1996;**16**: 250–3
6   Screnci D, Hirsch E, Levy K, Skawinski E, DerBoghosian M. Medical outreach to Armenia by telemedicine linkage. *J Med Syst* 1996;**20**:67–76
7   Treloar LL. Facts about teleconferencing for staff development administrators. *J Contin Educ Nurs* 1985;**16**:47–52
8   Herman CM, Buerki RA. Continuing professional education via radio: a review of the literature. *Am J Pharm Educ* 1977;**41**:192–5
9   Thornton RN. Nursing school of the air. *Aust Nurses J* 1986;**16**:50
10 Savela E, Enlund H. Public radio as a means of continuing education in pharmacy. *Am J Pharm Educ* 1996;**60**:374–7
11 Kaufman DM, Brock H. Enhancing interaction using videoconferencing in continuing health education. *J Contin Educ Health Prof* 1998;**18**:81–5
12 Fairbanks J, Viens D. Distance education for nurse practitioners: a partial solution. *J Am Acad Nurse Pract* 1995;**7**:499–503
13 Devaney S, Peterson SJ, Martin LK, Collier C. Continuing health education via interactive television: a pilot project. *J Nurs Staff Dev* 1996;**12**:98–100
14 Sanborn DE, Sanborn CJ, Seibert DJ, Welsh GW, Pike HF. Continuing education for nurses via interactive closed-circuit television: a pilot study. *Nurs Res* 1973;**22**:448–51
15 Hunter AT, Portis B. Medical educational television survey. *J Med Educ* 1972;**47**:57–63
16 Clark CE. Telecourses for nursing staff development. *J Nurse Staff Dev* 1989;**5**:107–10

17 Stephens HJ. Doctor to doctor via CCTV: continuing medical education in Louisiana. *Educ Ind Tv* 1974;**6**:11–14

18 Young HL. Medical education by satellite: the EuroTransMed experience. *J Audiov Media Med* 1995;**18**:75–8

19 Chouinard J. Satellite contributions to telemedicine: Canadian CME experiences. *Can Med Assoc J* 1983;**128**:850–5

20 McCauley J, Jenckes MW, McNutt LA. ASSERT: the effectiveness of a continuing medical education video on knowledge and attitudes about interpersonal violence. *Acad Med* 2003;**78**:518–24

21 Kripalani S, Cooper HP, Weinberg AD, Laufman L. Computer-assisted self-directed learning: the future of continuing medical education. *J Contin Educ Health Prof* 1997;**17**:114–20

22 Casebeer L, Bennett N, Kristofco R, Carillo A, Centor R. Physician Internet medical information seeking and on-line continuing education use patterns. *J Contin Educ Health Prof* 2002;**22**:33–42

23 Barnes BE. Creating the practice-learning environment: using information technology to support a new model of continuing medical education. *Acad Med* 1998;**73**:278–81

24 Sklar B. *The Current Status of Online CME*. Masters thesis, University of California, San Francisco, 2001. Available from http://www.cmelist.com/mastersthesis/ (last checked 25 June 2005)

25 Sikorski R, Peters R. Tools for change: CME on the Internet. *JAMA* 1998;**280**:1013–14

26 Potempa K, Stanley J, Davis B, Miller KL, Hassett MR, Pepicello S. Survey of distance technology use in AACN member schools. *J Prof Nurs* 2001;**17**:7–13

27 Carriere MF, Harvey D. Current state of distance continuing medical education in North America. *J Contin Educ Health Prof* 2001;**21**:150–7

28 Curran VR, Kirby F, Wells L. Survey of distance learning provision in continuing health professional education in Canada. *Can J Univ Contin Educ* 2003;**29**:51–72

29 Zollo SA, Kienzle MG, Henshaw Z, Crist LG, Wakefield DS. Tele-education in a telemedicine environment: implications for rural health care and academic medical centers. *J Med Syst* 1999;**23**:107–22

Further information

1 *Distance Education Clearinghouse* is a comprehensive and widely recognized Website that brings together distance education information from state, national and international sources (http://www.uwex.edu/disted/home.html).

2 *Distance Education at a Glance* provides a helpful overview of distance education for teachers, administrators, facilitators and students (http://www.uidaho.edu/eo/distglan.html).

3 *Online CME* includes an extensive listing of links to, and descriptions of, nearly 300 Websites offering more than 13,000 courses and more than 23,000 hours of CME credit (http://www.cmelist.com/).

4 *Conferencing on the Web* is a comprehensive index of tools and resources inthe area of online communication, including conferencing, collaborative work, e-learning and online communities. Both commercial and freeware tools are covered (http://thinkofit.com/webconf/).

Section 3: How to be Successful at Telemedicine

▶6

Defining the needs of a telemedicine service

Gary C Doolittle and Ryan J Spaulding

Introduction

The last decade has witnessed a rapid increase in telemedicine-related research and operational telemedicine programmes (see Chapter 1).[1] Yet, despite the growing interest in the field, it is difficult to ascertain the level of telemedicine activity that exists. This is because it is not easy to define what is, and what is not, telemedicine. In addition, numerous individuals and organizations practise telemedicine but would not consider themselves to have a dedicated telemedicine programme, and are not particularly enthusiastic about publicizing their efforts. The growing popularity of PC-based desktop videoconferencing for telemedicine will undoubtedly further this trend, making it even more difficult to define with any certainty the volume of telemedicine that is being done. Furthermore, telemedicine is teeming with politicians and self-appointed 'experts', speaking with apparent authority and offering volumes of advice, some of which is unfortunately based on extremely limited telemedicine experience, but which suggests that there may be more telemedicine activity than is actually the case.

Despite the difficulty of identifying and measuring telemedicine activity, industry profiles suggest that the number and size of programmes are increasing. The success or failure of these endeavours will undoubtedly have a significant effect on whether or not telemedicine becomes a part of mainstream health care in the future. For this reason, it is imperative that efforts are made to learn from the struggles and successes of first-generation programmes. This is particularly important considering the commonly experienced difficulty in sustaining telemedicine programmes after the initial set-up phase. For example, despite the effect that telemedicine is having on the health-care industry, many programmes rely on outside funding sources. In addition, few offer multiple telemedicine services or carry out large numbers of consultations. A 2001 study[2] conducted in the US by the Association of Telehealth Service Providers indicated that 48,000 teleconsultations were conducted across 82 reporting telemedicine programmes in the year 2000 (i.e. an average of only 585 consultations per programme per year). This is interesting in view of the attention that the field is receiving.

This chapter outlines areas that must be addressed when considering if telemedicine has anything to offer in a particular area of health service delivery and, once decided, when to initiate the telemedicine service. The approach involves defining the needs of a telemedicine application, as this is a fundamental requirement for developing a successful, sustainable service. The following recommendations are based on 14 years' experience of providing telemedicine services from the Kansas University Center for Telemedicine and Tele-health (KUCTT). In 1991, the KUCTT was one of only four active telemedicine providers in North America; in 2004 it was one of several hundred. In 1991, the KUCTT conducted a handful of consultations; in 2004, it conducted over 3200. Consultations occurred in hospitals, KU outreach offices, elementary schools, long-term care facilities, community mental health centres and even a children's day-care facility.

A telemedicine framework

The following steps outline a framework for defining the needs of a telemedicine service. The framework is designed to be generalizable to a variety of applications, and considers the needs of both consumers and providers. In what follows, a 'remote site' is one that receives telemedicine services, and a 'hub site' is one that delivers a telemedicine service (Figure 6.1).

Step 1. Defining the need for a telemedicine service
Many people do not have access to the health services they require to meet their individual clinical needs. This results in major disparities in measures of health status between and within countries. There are many reasons for this failure to meet health needs, which include economic and political factors. In the

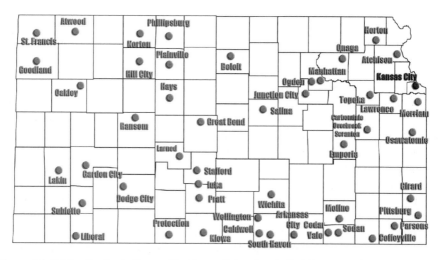

Figure 6.1 Telehealth sites in Kansas. The Kansas University Medical Center on the eastern edge of the state is the hub site and serves the other remote sites (Courtesy of the KUCTT)

industrialized world, another major consideration is geographical isolation or remoteness from centres where specialized services are available. For example, tertiary or secondary hospitals may have a rural referral base that traditionally necessitates patient travel to receive specialty care. In some instances, this has been partly addressed by specialists providing an intermittent 'outreach' clinic service. Even if this is the case – and certainly for those communities that never have any specialist services provided locally – the result is inequitable access to specialized services for those in rural communities compared with those living close to centres of specialized expertise. Expecting patients or highly skilled health-care workers to travel, often long distances, is a less than perfect situation. However, remoteness, which can result in a reduced quality of care, clearly represents an area of clinical need that should be addressed.

The important point when defining the needs of a telemedicine service is that a 'bottom-up' approach is essential. In other words, a deficient area of health care must be identified, rather than being invented by someone ready to try out a new system of health delivery or a technological development. Unfortunately, the most frequent error is to develop a telemedicine programme based on a new technology. Or, worse still, a funding source is identified, equipment is purchased, and only after implementation begins are the users consulted about their needs. Several years ago, the state mental health agencies in Kansas invested in 128 kbit/s desktop videoconferencing units to create a statewide infrastructure for psychiatric care. Today, the majority of these units sit idle, highlighting an initiative that overestimated technology's role in the diffusion of telemedicine. The important lesson from this is that programme design driven by technological imperatives is a recipe for failure.

Health-care workers who are in the business of delivering services, or consumers who are receiving them, are the people best placed to identify areas of deficiency within their locality. In any venture to improve health service delivery by telemedicine, such people should be consulted in detail at an early stage. After all of the above issues have been considered – and only then – should planning for an operational telemedicine service be initiated.

Step 2. Planning a service

The most significant decisions in programme development occur in the planning phase. Ideally, a telemedicine programme will align with the institutional goals, both clinical and business, of all participants. Determining the organizational strategy at this point is highly dependent on environmental factors, as well as organizational strengths and limitations.

Participants at the remote site are essential during the planning phase to ensure that the programme is developed from the 'bottom up'. A cohesive team must be built that includes physicians, nurses, technicians, information technologists and hospital administrators. In this fashion, development will take a grass roots approach, which will place the burden of success and failure on the population being served. Programme success is further enhanced when clinicians at the remote sites champion these efforts. Yellowlees[3] described this process as taking the 'bottom-up' approach to programme development. In referring to the importance of clinician drivers, he explained that:

> In recent years, there has tended to be the development of centralized 'project teams' in health departments. These teams generally lack both clinical expertise and practical telemedicine experience. In my experience, the teams in Australia tend to have broad, non-specific agendas covering wide ranges, specialties, needs, groups and geographical areas; they tend to concentrate on policy before practice. They are good at arranging technical demonstrations, but are bad at promoting the actual clinical use of telemedicine.

Clearly, developers must recognize the significant role of the rural clinicians when planning a telemedicine programme. While patients' needs are often the primary focus of a telemedicine endeavour, local clinicians' needs and interests must also be considered since they are the primary referral sources of patients to telemedicine clinics. In a recently completed Kansas study, Spaulding *et al.*[4] found that rural providers were more likely to make telemedicine referrals if they recognized an advantage to themselves in utilizing the telemedicine service. The salient lesson here is that telemedicine programmes cannot force remote sites to use their services. And frankly, the degree to which programmes can *influence* participation of the remote sites is grossly overestimated. Without local participation, telemedicine programmes are doomed to fail.

Programme focus and magnitude are additional critical issues when planning a programme. It is easy to become overenthusiastic about the potential of telemedicine applications. However, it is generally best to err on the side of caution when starting new ventures. If demand is overestimated, attenuation of services may be viewed negatively and may impede progress in other areas.

An effective, though not always foolproof strategy, is to plan carefully for a new service and build on those projects that prove themselves successful. This was illustrated in the KUCTT school-based telemedicine project called TeleKidcare (Figure 6.2). Preparing to launch this school-based service took almost a year. Frequent meetings were held between members of a planning team composed of nurses, educators, telemedicine administrative staff and physicians. The initial TeleKidcare pilot trial enjoyed great success. The clinical demand grew and multiple physicians were invited to participate in the second year. It was interesting to observe a decline in the number of requested consultations as the number of providers increased. School nurses cited a lack of continuity and comfort level with new physicians as causes for the fall in referrals. Notably, this was the only time in the project when consultations did not increase from month to month. This experience illustrates the need to balance the number of providers in a system with the maturation of the project. The TeleKidcare clinical director now requires formal training of paediatricians – including training sessions with school-based nurses – prior to participation in the service. Furthermore, all her paediatric residents participate in the school-based project, which provides valuable training experience and prepares future telehealth providers for telemedicine.

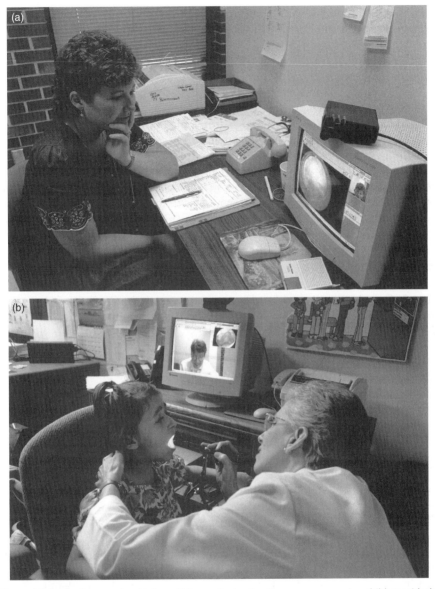

Figure 6.2 In the Kansas school telemedicine project, school nurses can examine children with the benefit of expertise from the KUMC: (a) consultation with paediatrician; (b) examination of the child's mouth. (Photo credit: KUCTT)

Telemedical services must also be grounded in a sound business plan for the project to be launched and sustained. However, several issues can complicate an organization's plans. An important philosophical issue to consider is the nature of the working relationship, *real and perceived*, with the remote sites. For example, rural hospital administrators often view telemedicine as offering competing rather than complementary services, viewing telemedicine as a mechanism for larger health facilities to attract patients from the local region. For this reason, hub sites that partner with remote sites by keeping patients within the local health-care system may improve the chances of a sustainable telemedicine programme. However, from an administrative perspective, this may not be feasible if the capital outlay for the equipment, technician time and availability, and maintenance fees are borne by the hub site. As programmes set goals to reach rural areas, the organizational mission must be carefully balanced in order to bring about a 'win–win' situation for both sites.

A good example of a complementary service based on a 'cost-saving' business plan comes from the Kansas telemedicine programme. In Kansas, there are fewer than 10 paediatric cardiologists, most of whom are located in Kansas City or Wichita, leaving many rural *and* urban areas without access to this sub-specialty. By using existing videoconferencing equipment at a medium-sized hospital in central Kansas, physicians there are able to transmit live echocardiograms to paediatric cardiologists at the Kansas University Medical Center. The use of existing equipment avoids the need for an expensive initial investment.

Step 3. Conducting a needs assessment

In addition to the measures outlined in step 1, developers must also assess the needs for the telemedicine service from a clinical, economic and technical perspective.

Clinical

From a clinical perspective, it is important to remember that certain clinical services can be provided via telemedicine while others cannot. Furthermore, some areas of medicine (e.g. child psychiatry) adapt well to telemedical delivery, while others (e.g. surgical subspecialties) are more difficult, requiring more from the local practitioner. For example, even if a need for help in the management of high-risk pregnancy emerges, the clinicians with skills to manage these patients, coupled with their remote counterparts, may not feel comfortable about providing this service by telemedicine. Clinical needs for each potential telemedicine site must be analysed separately, given that each has a different complement of practitioners possessing specific talents, perhaps having trained in different areas. Clearly, a small rural community with a sole family medicine physician will offer very different clinical services compared to a secondary health-care facility with multiple specialists on staff. These challenges are compounded when clinicians have little or no prior knowledge or experience of telemedicine.

By meeting with remote physicians, nurses and hospital administrators, an assessment of the local health-care delivery system can be conducted. Face-to-face meetings allow the interest and enthusiasm of the local providers to be assessed. It is important to determine what the remote health-care community perceives as the benefits of telemedicine. A description of the services that are performed at the remote site is necessary, giving an idea of the local health-care

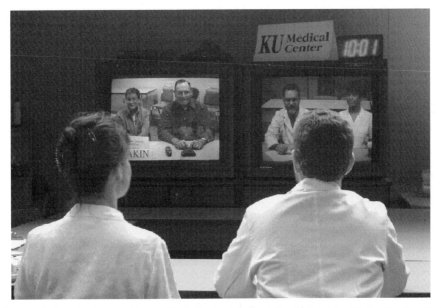

Figure 6.3 Oncologist consulting with a patient, with the patient's daughter joining the physician for the meeting (Photo credit: KUCTT)

infrastructure as well as the training and skill level of the practitioners. Surveys and interviews with providers (focus groups) are techniques that will reveal services for which patients are routinely referred from the local district and are therefore candidates for telemedicine. Such research should primarily target remote physicians because they understand local health-care needs and will have insights into the applications that will be best served telemedically. By including the clinicians in this process, programme developers take the first steps in building a team with the remote community. If staff at the remote site are not comfortable about receiving certain services via telemedicine, the project will not succeed. For example, in a tele-oncology clinic (Figure 6.3) the diagnosis of cancer may be made only to find that the remote physician is unwilling to manage the side-effects of chemotherapy, or that the nursing staff are not trained in chemotherapy administration. If the local infrastructure cannot support the requested service, the remote participants must decide whether they wish to develop it. Using the above example, when oncology services are requested, it is essential for remote nurses to be competent in chemotherapy administration if patients are to remain at home. Perhaps the hub site will offer chemotherapy administration training, allowing members from both sites to meet, fostering the team-building process.

Economic
Telemedicine programme developers must assess needs from an economic perspective and hospital administrators are normally essential participants in

Table 6.1 Tele-oncology clinic costs for 121 consultations (from Doolittle et al.[5])

	Actual cost (US$)
Kansas University Medical Center	
Technology	
Telemedicine room/equipment	612
Technician expense	2,643
Technology subtotal	3,255
Practice expenses	
Scheduler expense	2,096
Fax/telephone	381
Office rent	332
Network access	113
Office practice subtotal	2,922
KUMC subtotal	6,177
Hays Medical Center	
Technology	
Telemedicine room	364
Telemedicine equipment*	1,194
Equipment maintenance[†]	1,750
Technician time	1,525
Telecommunication line charges	3,600
Technology subtotal	8,433
Practice expenses	
Physician contract	18,000
Nursing staff salary	7,684
Secretarial staff salaries	7,758
Billing expenses	660
Fax/telephone	242
Transcription service	710
Office practice subtotal	35,054
HMC subtotal	43,487
Total	*49,664*
Cost per visit	*410*

*Depreciated cost
[†]Some equipment maintenance was done under contract and is listed under telemedicine equipment and technician

this process. As part of this approach, it is useful to consider start-up and maintenance expenses, as well as potential revenue streams. Implementation costs may be categorized as personnel- or technology-related expenses.[4] Funds for the technology must cover hardware and software, peripheral devices and equipment maintenance for both sites. Personnel, including nursing staff and technical support staff, must be identified at both remote and hub sites. Based on the projected patient workload, staffing time must be estimated as well as telecommunication use and expenses. As an example, actual cost data from a tele-oncology clinic are shown in Table 6.1.[5] The average cost was $410 per patient, which was significantly lower than in a study five years before, which found an average cost of $816 per patient.[6]

During the programme design stage, a decision should be made about how start-up and maintenance costs will be divided between sites. For example, the telecommunication line charges may be borne by either or both sites. If the remote site provides a consistent referral stream, the hub site may be willing to pay the telecommunication charges; or the remote hospital may agree to pay programme-related expenses since telemedicine enables patient evaluations and treatment to take place locally, thus bringing revenues from services that would have been provided elsewhere. For other forms of telemedicine (e.g. teleradiology or telecardiology), reimbursement for services will be attractive to hospital administrators and clinicians at both sites.

A primary concern is the need for programmes to assess, and in some cases, *negotiate* reimbursement practices for professional services. Providers will insist on some form of compensation for professional services rendered. Reimbursement has often been identified as an impediment to the diffusion of telemedicine, although Lapolla and Millis[7] have argued that this issue has been exaggerated out of all proportion. This is even more likely now that widely expanded reimbursement is available via Medicare, as well as through Medicaid in at least 22 states. In Kansas, for example, the Blue Cross/Blue Shield organization has considerable flexibility with regard to payment, and in fact was one of the first organizations in the US to pay for teleconsultations. Telemedicine became reimbursable by the three largest insurers in Kansas in August 2004.

Despite the challenges of reimbursement, alternative funding sources may be sought to cover telemedicine services. Identifying funding streams and developing contracts for services is one way to ensure compensation for teleconsultations. The best example of this model occurs in prison telemedicine. Contracts between telemedicine providers and correctional facilities ensure that inmates will be cared for, and at the same time obviate the need for travel away from prison, a significant operating expense.[8] Thus providers are compensated for their professional services while the prison saves transport-related expenses.

In the managed care model, fixed reimbursement is provided in exchange for medical services. In this system, the cost of care provided via telemedicine may be justified if telemedicine can be used to replace some in-person visits. Telehospice care illustrates this well. Traditional hospice care involves many home visits by nurses and social workers. In Kansas, this is particularly challenging as hospice providers must sometimes drive long distances to provide care for the rural sector. Telehospice – the use of home-based telemedicine units to conduct nursing and social work visits – was first used to reach rural patients in need of care at the end of life.[9] In this setting, telehospice care was designed to augment traditional in-home hospice care. A cost analysis revealed a large difference between expenses incurred from a telehospice visit ($29) and those from an in-person visit (over $120).[10] Thus it is easy for hospice administrators to justify telemedicine expenses, especially considering that, in the US, home-based hospice care is reimbursed on a fixed *per diem* basis under the Medicare Hospice Benefit.

The financial needs assessment should consider the expenses related to the patient population as well. Direct and indirect costs relating to travel are significant and frequently overlooked patient expenses. Direct expenses include fees for transportation, food and accommodation. Indirect costs, which are often substantial, include time off work for patients and family members, and even additional child-care costs incurred due to hub hospital visits. Telemedicine may avoid the need for travel, producing economic benefits for patients and family members. Programme developers may recognize this as one of the benefits, and should take advantage of the potential marketing value in a remote community.

During the economic needs assessment, a potential conflict of interest may surface. The administrator, driven by economics, may wish to keep the patient and services locally, while the primary care team may feel inadequately trained to provide care, even with the supervision of a telemedical specialist. In this situation, telemedicine could serve to raise the standard of care and to shift greater responsibility to the local health-care team. However, if the remote providers are unwilling to shoulder a higher level of responsibility, even if in the best financial interest of the remote site, a conflict may arise.

Technology

Technology issues must also be included in the needs assessment. In addition, an inventory of the technology available at all sites must be carried out. For example, videoconferencing systems may already be in use for educational purposes. These units may be readily adapted for teleconsultation. An understanding of the remote network infrastructure will be necessary to determine the best technological solution. Part of this process is to assess the bandwidth actually required for telemedicine – something that is frequently overestimated. In fact, at the KUMC, the most common bandwidth in use is 128 kbit/s, lower than that reported in other US telemedicine networks in the 1990s.[11]

In recent years, as high-speed Internet access has become more readily available in rural areas, telemedicine has become possible using computer networks and the Internet protocol (IP) instead of circuit-switched networks such as ISDN. This eliminates hourly line charges when a telemedicine connection is made and can also deliver videoconferencing to any location that has a PC with Internet connectivity (see Chapter 2). This may make telemedicine cheaper and more convenient, which in turn may facilitate the growth of home telehealth activity. Although the use of IP transmission for telemedicine is promising, the security and quality of the connection requires significantly more attention than it does with digital lines. Internet lines are also more vulnerable to hacking. If the telemedicine connection travels through the public Internet, it may be subject to bandwidth limitations, causing poor video or audio quality and making the teleconsultation unsatisfactory. Because of these issues, using the public Internet for telemedicine is not recommended at present.

The selection of peripheral devices should also be needs-driven. For example, for the school-based telemedicine project, a digital otoscope and electronic stethoscope were deemed essential by both paediatricians and school nurses.[12] Alternatively, when planning for a teleoncology practice, the stethoscope was considered essential, as was a document camera enabling the consultant to review computerized tomography scans online as part of the evaluation.[13] However, for adult and child telepsychiatry services, peripheral devices are not normally required. While it is best to let the clinicians who provide the expertise determine what peripheral devices are required at the remote sites, telemedicine developers must encourage clinicians to be flexible about their perceived requirements. For instance, an internist who routinely examines the ears and throat of a patient may come to rely on the on-site practitioner's examination during a teleconsultation, obviating the need for an electronic otoscope.

Other considerations

Reorganization is another important consideration when planning for telemedicine services and will be highly dependent on the technologies being considered. For example, desktop videoconferencing units generally occupy less space than room-based units and may be housed in doctors' offices as opposed to clinic areas. The telecommunications medium chosen will also affect the organizational structure. Funding issues further complicate matters. If a programme has limited financial support, outside sources may be sought to fund programme development, personnel, marketing and evaluation activities. This may result in jobs and particular activities being shared by sites that are not working together in the same health-care delivery system. This requires forming partnerships that may not have existed previously.

The appropriateness of organizational and technological infrastructures should be a primary concern of programme developers. In addition, the strategy should address ergonomic issues for both caregivers and patients. A simple step such as locating the telemedicine equipment in close proximity to the providers may have a significant effect on the adoption and functioning of a programme. If a unit is placed in another building or on a different floor, then the probability of its use is lower.

Step 4. Developing a health-care team

While 'team development' is generally described as the process of turning a collection of individuals into a group which identifies itself as a team, both the nature of the process (team building) and the end product (teams) are variously defined.[14-16] Similar confusion exists when discussing telemedicine teams. Are we referring to individuals at remote sites exclusively? Should teams be restricted only to the caregivers, perhaps both at the remote and distant locations? Or do teams encompass a much broader group, including administrators, schedulers, technicians, patients and even family members of patients in some cases?

There is no simple answer to these questions. For this reason, developing a health-care team is an essential, yet difficult, step in building a successful telemedicine programme. It is complicated by several factors. Organizations are likely to have different values and missions. Therefore, the organizational philosophies driving services may also be different. Team members may have conflicting roles and functions. For example, someone coordinating room and provider schedules will have a tendency to place great importance on punctuality. In contrast, technicians usually view service issues from a technological perspective, while physicians are primarily interested in the clinical outcome. All of these issues are further complicated when the parties are geographically dispersed throughout a region or state.

The members of the telemedicine team must be identified through the needs assessment process. At the remote site members will include physicians, nurses, videoconferencing technicians and possibly a hospital administrator. At the hub site, the team may consist of the consultant physician, nurse, technician and scheduler. The relationship between the consultant physician and the presenter is critical to the success of any telemedicine project. In Kansas, the presenter is usually a nurse, depending on the service being provided and assuming that the problem is routine. The on-site presenter is essential for the successful practice of telemedicine. While the primary care physician at the remote site is a welcome participant, he or she may not have time to be present for a tele-medicine consultation. However, if the patient is seriously ill and requires an urgent consultation, the local physician may choose to be present to facilitate a rapid evaluation and a prompt treatment plan. Therefore, it is essential for the consultant physician to develop a positive working relationship with the nurse or the other presenter. Initially, some presenters find it awkward to have their assessments directly observed by the consultant and stressful to remember that the specialist is relying on that assessment and physical examination to make a decision. Given time, however, a positive working relationship between consultant and presenter should develop, which will enhance the service. As in traditional practice, physician-to-physician relationships and communication must develop to ensure success. If a good working relationship develops between the primary care physician and the physician consultant, referrals to the telemedicine clinic will continue. At the KUCTT, the scheduler has played a significant role in facilitating communication between team members, including physicians, nurses and technicians.

Programme developers must recognize the significant role of the remote team in sustaining services. Without a strong supporting cast at the remote location, telemedicine programmes rarely succeed. Unfortunately, programmes rarely recognize the significant role of remote teams in this process. This message is reinforced as recognition is frequently directed at hub sites and consultant providers, and only rarely includes the local caregivers. In reality, the 'medicine' of 'telemedicine' occurs at the remote site, and, without a strong local care team, the telemedicine process will fail. It is essential for the staff at the remote site to be recognized as integral members of the team. Some effective ways to build teams are discussed below.

Step 5. Marketing

Despite the growth of telemedicine applications, the barriers facing new programmes should not be underestimated. Reimbursement and liability concerns exemplify a few of these challenges. Programmes are constantly faced with justifying their existence and are often teetering on the brink of going out of business. For this reason, a significant effort should be dedicated to marketing services. This also serves a secondary purpose because telemedicine practice often requires participants to take on new roles (i.e. a nurse serving as the case presenter and on-site examiner). Taking on new roles may be associated with considerable unease, making it easier for new team members to revert to traditional practices when operational difficulties surface. Marketing, from this perspective, is as much an internal as it is an external function. Telemedicine programmes must constantly remind team members of their importance, and of the significance of services provided. For example, in the school-based project at the KUCTT, school nurses attend monthly meetings serving practical, emotional and social needs. Paediatric physicians attend the meetings, as well as administrative and technical staff from the KUCTT. These meetings serve an important team-building function for all of the participants in the project.

Marketing practices add to programme sustainability by enhancing current services and creating future opportunities. For example, the telepsychiatrists at the KUCTT are well known throughout the state of Kansas for their telemedicine work. As a result, their services are frequently requested, either for one-off consultation or for continuing evaluation and management. While the practice originally involved the south-eastern part of the state, psychiatric consultations have now been performed at multiple sites all across the state. What started as a service for one community mental health centre has grown into a full telepsychiatry practice, with services provided in a variety of different contexts, including a day care centre, hospitals, a juvenile detention centre and a shelter for battered women.

Step 6. Evaluating the programme

Evaluating a telemedicine programme should be viewed as an integral step in programme design and implementation, and is discussed in detail in Chapter 8. Results of a formal evaluation process will provide feedback to participants and enable the decision-makers to assess the current and future direction of the programme. The fact that members from different health-care teams are involved will complicate the evaluation process. For example, one site may define effectiveness in terms of access to services while another may measure success by cost savings. From the policy-maker's perspective, access to care may be considered most important, even if the telemedicine project is unable to sustain itself financially from the generation of clinical revenues. The hub site may measure success in terms of patients who are referred to that facility. This may be further complicated if the value added is addressed from the patients' perspective. There may be considerable cost savings if travel is avoided, but this is not always an expense that is borne by the health-care system.

Conclusion

The framework discussed in this chapter should be used as a guide for planning new telemedicine programmes. While programme objectives, technologies and even philosophies will differ (sometimes tremendously), certain common factors that enhance programme success can be identified. A key factor is the ability of the developers to recognize that the concepts that make people excited about telemedicine – namely the integration of new technologies and medicine – should not be the concepts that drive organizational strategy. Unfortunately, there are numerous examples of telemedicine projects that have failed because technology was used as the driving force for change, before it had been established that there was a deficiency in health-care delivery or that there was a desire to address it. The success of future telemedicine programmes will be strongly related to their ability to recognize that they should be used to enhance current health-care delivery rather than to replace it.

References

1   Taylor P. A survey of research in telemedicine. 1: Telemedicine systems. *J Telemed Telecare* 1998;**4**:1–17
2   Dahlin MP, Wachter G, Engle WM, Henderson J. *2001 Report on U.S. Telemedicine Activity.* Portland, OR: Association of Telehealth Service Providers, 2001
3   Yellowlees P. Successful development of telemedicine systems – seven core principles. *J Telemed Telecare* 1997;**3**:215–6
4   Spaulding RJ, Russo T, Cook DJ, Doolittle GC. Diffusion theory and telemedicine adoption by Kansas health-care providers: critical factors in telemedicine adoption for improved patient access. *J Telemed Telecare* 2005;**11** (Suppl. 1):107–9
5   Doolittle GC, Williams AR, Spaulding A, Spaulding RJ, Cook DJ. A cost analysis of a tele-oncology practice in the United States. *J Telemed Telecare* 2004;**10**:27–9
6   Doolittle GC, Williams A, Harmon A, *et al.* A cost measurement study for a tele-oncology practice. *J Telemed Telecare* 1998;**4**:84–8
7   Lapolla M, Millis B. Is telemedicine reimbursement a real barrier or a convenient straw man? *Telemed Today* 1997;**5**(6):5
8   McCue MJ, Mazmanian PE, Hampton C, *et al.* The case of Powhatan Correctional Center/Virginia Department of Corrections and Virginia Commonwealth University/Medical College of Virginia. *Telemed J* 1997;**3**:11–17
9   Doolittle GC, Yaezel A, Otto F, Clemens C. Hospice care using home-based telemedicine systems. *J Telemed Telecare* 1998;**4** (Suppl. 1):58–9
10 Doolittle GC. A cost measurement study for a home-based telehospice service. *J Telemed Telecare* 2000;**6** (Suppl. 1):193–5
11 Allen A, Wheeler T. The leaders: US programs doing more than 500 interactive consults in 1997. *Telemed Today* 1998;**6**(3):36–7
12 Whitten P, Cook DJ, Shaw P, Ermer D, Goodwin J. TelekidCare: bringing health care into schools. *Telemed J* 1999;**4**:335–43
13 Doolittle GC, Allen A. Practising oncology via telemedicine. *J Telemed Telecare* 1997;**3**:63–70
14 Parker PK, Woodruff D. Reliability and validity of the Parker team player survey. *Educ Psychol Meas* 1994;**54**:1030–7
15 Larson CE, LaFasto FMJ. *Teamwork.* Newbury Park, CA: Sage, 1989
16 Buller BF, Bell CH. Effects of team building and goal setting on productivity: a field experiment. *Acad Manage J* 1986;**29**:305–28

Further information

1   Walker J, Whetton S. The diffusion of innovation: factors influencing the uptake of telehealth. *J Telemed Telecare* 2002;**8** (Suppl. 3):73–5
2   Gagnon MP, Lamothe L, Fortin JP, *et al.* Telehealth adoption in hospitals: an organisational perspective. *J Health Organ Manage* 2005;**19**:32–56
3   Menachemi N, Burke DE, Ayers DJ. Factors affecting the adoption of telemedicine – a multiple adopter perspective. *J Med Syst* 2004;**28**:617–32

Successfully developing a telemedicine system

Peter M Yellowlees

Introduction

We live in a changing world. It has been suggested (following work by Mercedes-Benz) that 12-year-olds can drive a car better using paddles, such as are used for Nintendo games, than adults using steering wheels. It is entirely possible that in 20 or 30 years the steering wheel may be of purely historical interest as the way we drive cars – if cars still exist – changes over time.

Successfully developing telemedicine systems is primarily about effective change management within an already rapidly changing health-care environment. Unfortunately, there are many examples around the world where telemedicine has been introduced and rapidly abandoned, often because it has simply not been integrated into the surrounding health and business environment. Charismatic clinicians have typically started telemedicine programmes and have convinced funding authorities to give them often very substantial amounts of money for interesting applications, but the projects have then failed when the project money ran out, or the individual clinicians lost interest, energy or direction. As a consequence, many expensive telemedicine systems have lain idle and eventually been discarded after relatively little use.

The costs of failing to introduce a telemedicine system properly are enormous. These comprise not only the financial costs of the equipment and time put into the development, but perhaps more importantly the long-term psychological costs of failure. One project failing in a high-profile area can destroy the reputation of telemedicine as a potential health-care delivery system over a very much wider area. Also, a failed telemedicine system that simply remains in place, unused, yet too expensive to discard immediately, is a constant reminder to clinicians and administrators alike of the unsuccessful project. Inevitably, in these situations, the whole practice of telemedicine itself attracts an unenviable reputation, and it may be years before another attempt is made to provide telemedicine services in a region where telemedicine has failed once already.

After the early telemedicine experiments in the 1960s and 1970s, and after the majority of projects ended in failure, a widespread psychological turnoff from telemedicine occurred. Very little telemedicine was done during the 1980s and it was not until prices came down and technology improved in the 1990s that telemedicine systems were rediscovered by a new generation of enthusiasts, who had not had poor experiences during the first phase of telemedicine experimentation. In the new millennium, with the advent of the Internet and broadband networks, and in part driven by military and defence applications, telemedicine has become much more firmly established internationally than it ever was in the 1960s and 1970s. It is crucial that it does not fail as a health delivery system once more. We must learn from history that the major single lesson when implementing telemedicine systems is that they must be integrated into the health-care environment.

Nearly a decade ago, Smith[1] described what he termed 'the future of health-care systems' where information technology and consumerism will transform health care worldwide. He commented that most sectors of industrialized economies, such as transport, manufacturing and telecommunications, have been transformed in the past 20 years, whereas health care has not. He described a view of the future where health care will be provided through both integrated and virtual systems, anywhere, anytime, and where clinicians will focus on long-term relationships with patients, suppliers, funders and insurers, with the patient's role being much greater and more assertive than at present. Smith predicted that 'industrial age medicine' will invert to become 'information age health care', where, 'instead of being viewed as the apex of a system of care that hardly recognizes the large amount of self-care that occurs now, professional care will be viewed as a support to a system that emphasizes self-care' (Figure 7.1).

Why is a futuristic perspective important when developing telemedicine systems? Simply because such systems will make a dramatic difference to the health-care environment as we know it today. While Smith and others look at the future of health care and see huge changes, the present reality is that, at the beginning of the 21st century, the business of health care remains essentially as a multitude of small cottage industries, powerful autocratic empires or mysterious, protected and poorly defined systems that often not even the clinicians who work within them can understand. While many new technologies, such as telephones, fax machines, tape recorders, televisions and computers, have been gradually accepted and used by doctors over the last few decades, the average doctor still works in a way that has changed remarkably little over the past 30 years. In some respects, the way that many health-care information systems have been introduced has actually had a negative effect on clinicians, as they have often been seen to be a tool of management, concentrating mainly on costs or on restricting clinicians' practice. All this does is to alienate clinicians further, and make them less likely to be interested in clinically useful tools within the telemedicine field.

All of these changes are upon us, and many of them will overtake us shortly. Also, they all have to be thoroughly understood in order to implement telemedicine systems in the changing environment of health care. Many clinicians are ready to embrace these changes, but many others are not. Many health-care systems and services are interested in moving forward and adapting, while others prefer to die, or to remain uncompetitive and slowly bleed away over the years until they are beyond rehabilitation. Many information technology and telemedicine industry members simply see health care as a fatted calf to be milked rapidly for short-term profit, instead of looking at the longer-term collaborative

Industrial age medicine

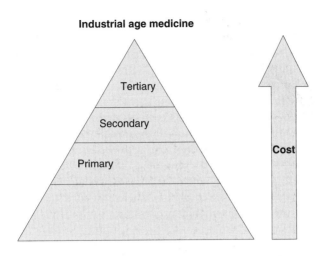

Information age health care

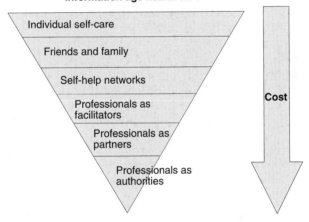

Figure 7.1 The transformation from industrial age medicine to health care in the information age (based on Smith[1])

unions that can be created with health-care providers to the benefit of both. Finally, and most important, many patients remain ignorant of their ability, and power, to influence change within the health sector, either individually or through the various national political processes around the world. If only because of its cost, health is becoming increasingly important politically, and the changes that invite much greater use of telemedicine in the future will, if they are not driven from within the health-care system, be driven externally by these political forces.

These changes are beginning to occur. Nowhere are telemedicine and information technology potentially more critical in the redesign of the health-care delivery systems than in rural and frontier areas,[2] where they have the potential to change dramatically the way that health care occurs. As Smith predicted, we are starting to move from health-care systems aimed at providing episodic, institutional care for the treatment of illnesses, to information-based systems that seek to promote increased consumer and carer involvement in the prevention of illness across the lifespan. With the advent of the Internet and broadband networks, health care is gradually becoming a distributed information industry in many metropolitan and some rural areas.

Over the past few decades, there has been an explosion in new science, leading to a better understanding of medicine and the mechanisms of disease. The need to manage this information and rapidly bring it to the point of care has led the call for increased use of information technology in health care.[3,4] The Institute of Medicine report *Crossing the Quality Chasm* stated that information technology 'must play a central role in the redesign of the health-care system'.[5] Telemedicine should be at the front of this change process.

Barriers to telemedicine implementation

Treister has examined why clinicians often fail to accept new information systems.[6] He quotes 11 reasons, as shown in Table 7.1. All of Treister's reasons apply to telemedicine systems and all must be taken into account when designing them. All of these issues can certainly be addressed and overcome. I described seven core principles in successfully developing a telemedicine system in 1997[7] and these are updated in Table 7.2. I have updated the principles as follows:

Principle 1: Telemedicine applications and sites should be selected pragmatically, rather than philosophically

The general experience of telemedicine is that it will fail if there are not clinicians and other users at all sites who are interested in using the technique for the benefit of patients and themselves. Unfortunately, there are many examples around the world of telemedicine systems having being introduced into health-care environments where there is no support, interest or skill to use them, but where there is a clear potential need. Unfortunately, these systems tend to remain packed in their boxes, unopened and unused. If unwilling clinicians are forced to use

Table 7.1 Reasons why physicians fail to accept new information systems (Treister[6])

1.	Too much change ('change toxicity')
2.	Failure to begin with an adequate physician base of support
3.	Lack of a user-friendly interface
4.	Concern regarding the information collected
5.	Failure to collect the most important information
6.	Physician technophobia
7.	Excluding physician involvement from the financial analysis
8.	Failure to include marketing to physicians in the implementation plan
9.	Inadequate training of physicians to use the system
10.	Lack of strong, centralized information systems leadership respected by physicians
11.	Lack of control by the organization over physician practices

Table 7.2 Principles for the successful development of telemedicine systems (adapted from Yellowlees[7])

1.	Telemedicine applications and sites should be selected pragmatically, rather than philosophically
2.	Clinician drivers and telemedicine users must own the systems
3.	Telemedicine management and support should follow best-practice business principles
4.	The technology should be as user-friendly as possible
5.	Telemedicine users must be well trained and supported, both technically and professionally
6.	Telemedicine applications should be evaluated and sustained in a clinically appropriate and user-friendly manner
7.	Information about the development of telemedicine must be shared

them, they can become a symbol of a 'big brother' approach to health care, and are seen as being both intrusive and useless, as well as suffering, mysteriously, multiple technical breakdowns and mishaps! It is much more sensible to identify active, interested clinicians within a health service, provide them with the telemedicine support for whatever is their specialty of interest, and let them act as telemedicine 'champions', gradually infecting other clinicians around them with their enthusiasm. As such, telemedicine enhances and improves existing health sciences, rather than being initially used to provide a service where none previously existed or, worse still, to replace a previous service.

Principle 2: Clinician drivers and telemedicine users must own the systems

The literature widely supports the importance of 'clinician drivers' or 'telemedicine champions' as being of vital significance. The key issue here is supporting these interested clinicians who are prepared to be innovative and dynamic in their use of telemedicine, to value them and to acknowledge their importance, and to involve them in as much of the planning of the organizational aspects of the telemedicine systems as is possible. Ownership is the key word. We all know, in our lives outside of medicine, that if we care about something, and feel pride and ownership in it, that we are going to look after it better, value it more and use it more effectively. Conversely, if we do not care about something, we do not tend to use it so well. Hence, within health care, if clinicians are to be innovative, to experiment, to evaluate and teach others about telemedicine, it is crucial for them to own the system.

Principle 3: Telemedicine management and support should follow best-practice business principles

While telemedicine is new for most clinicians, and frightening for some, the majority of clinicians are perfectly capable of becoming technically and clinically competent at performing telemedicine. There is therefore no need to introduce another layer of management, who might place bureaucratic controls on them. Both 'bottom up' and 'top down' management are required – neither on their own will suffice – rather than any special management approach that treats telemedicine like a 'special case' within the health environment. One particular development to be wary of is the formation of centralized 'project teams' in health departments with the purpose of driving telemedicine. Generally, these teams lack both clinical expertise and practical telemedicine experience. They may have broad, non-specific agendas covering wide ranges, specialties, needs, groups and geographical areas, and they tend to concentrate on policy before practice. They are good at arranging technical demonstrations, but are bad at promoting the actual clinical use of telemedicine. Such teams may exclude clinicians from decision making, either consciously or unconsciously, and often tend to become overconcerned about legal and confidentiality issues, probably because they do not have a good understanding of the real clinical world.

Principle 4: The technology should be as user-friendly as possible

Fortunately, there is a general move away from 'special telemedicine rooms', which are threatening and often inconvenient to clinicians, and tend to be locked, inaccessible, or depend on the presence of a technician to operate them. The future for telemedicine is simple computer-based systems that are located in, and integrated into, normal work environments, generally on the desktop, in association with other applications such as electronic record systems. Clinicians are busy people and it is often too much trouble, or time, to walk up several flights of stairs within the same building to find the telemedicine system, never mind going down the road to a different building (see Chapter 6 for further details). Interfaces are becoming much simpler and most systems are now being designed using Internet protocols, which allow more interactivity with other programmes and scheduling systems. Clinicians will certainly use technologies if they are available and clinician-friendly. If, however, they are inaccessible, or so complicated to use that it is constantly necessary to revise how to use them, then they will neither be supported nor used appropriately.

Principle 5: Telemedicine users must be well trained and supported, both technically and professionally

Training is vital. If a telemedicine programme is to have one motto that will ensure success, it should be 'Train, train and train again'. Such training can often take place quite unconsciously. For example, meetings and education sessions using telemedicine can be introduced early on in a telemedicine programme as a way of getting clinicians used to operating with videoconferencing and telemedicine systems in a normal health-care environment. As part of an audience where telemedicine is being used, clinicians can study the equipment, watch how it is operated, check that it is non-threatening and allay many of their anxieties, rather than having to confront all of the human and technical issues around telemedicine at once with their first use in a patient-related consultation. Once clinicians see telemedicine as part of their normal health-care environment, they mostly then start using it for clinical purposes on a voluntary basis. This 'silent' training has, naturally, to be supported by more formal training programmes, as described above.

Principle 6: Telemedicine applications should be evaluated and sustained in a clinically appropriate and user-friendly manner

There is still a great need for proper evaluations of telemedicine at a national and international level. How this can be done is described in Chapter 8. At the local level, when implementing a programme, another approach is to evaluate the effectiveness of the programme in the context of a business plan. Put simply, this involves assessing whether or not defined outcome measures have been achieved, within a reasonable time-frame, and with the input of appropriate resources, by implementing the programme. A business plan is different from a formal research protocol, although there are similarities in the two methods of assessment. Many early telemedicine programmes were not created with sustainability in mind, but telemedicine is now sufficiently well entrenched worldwide that the concept of financial sustainability should be incorporated at the earliest planning stage. Implementation of a new telemedicine programme using a business plan is more likely to make it sustainable over time, as it will ensure that the necessary equipment, staff costs and technical support are properly funded.

Principle 7: Information about the development of telemedicine must be shared

Unfortunately, there is still inadequate information about telemedicine based on the results of properly conducted scientific trials, although the evidence base for telemedicine is increasing and there are now a number of randomized controlled studies that support the practice in certain specialties, such as radiology, dermatology and psychiatry. Much of our present information is still based on historical polemic or idiosyncratic opinion. If telemedicine is to realize its full potential, it must be properly evaluated and the results of any evaluations published, whether those results are positive or negative (see Chapter 8). Since telemedicine is about communication with colleagues and patients across large distances, it should be possible for those involved in it to do the same with their experiences.

Conclusion

Developing a telemedicine service can be a daunting task. There are, however, many successful telemedicine services around the world, and it is crucial to learn from them. Solutions are generally available, and can be based on the principles defined in this and the previous chapter. There are, of course, many barriers, not the least of which are the cultural, legal and ethical ones that are discussed in Chapter 11. Implementing telemedicine requires an understanding of the health-care environment and a decision to integrate telemedicine within that environment. A process that involves good business planning, the involvement of a wide range of interested parties and support for clinician drivers, as well as strong corporate and political support, is likely to lead to long-term success. Speaking to, and learning from, one's colleagues will make that success even more certain, and evaluating the service, so as to prove its effectiveness, in a clinical and business sense, will ensure continuing political and financial support.

References

1   Smith R. The future of health care systems. *BMJ* 1997;**314**:1495–6
2   Institute of Medicine. *Quality Through Collaboration – The Future of Rural Health*. Washington, DC: National Academies Press, 2004
3   Glick TH, Moore GT. Time to learn: the outlook for renewal of patient-centred education in the digital age. *Med Educ* 2001;**35**:505–9
4   Smith R. What clinical information do doctors need? *BMJ* 1996;**313**:1062–8
5   Institute of Medicine. *Crossing the Quality Chasm: A New Health System for the 21st Century*. Washington, DC. National Academies Press, 2001
6   Treister NW. Physician acceptance of new medical information systems: the field of dreams. *Phys Exec* 1998;**24**:20–4
7   Yellowlees P. Successful development of telemedicine systems – seven core principles. *J Telemed Telecare* 1997;**3**:215–22

Further information

1   Whitten P, Cook D (eds). *Understanding Health Communication Technologies*. San Francisco: Jossey-Boss, 2004

▶8

Evaluating telemedicine systems and services

Paul Taylor

Introduction

Over the last 20 years an extraordinary number of articles have been written about telemedicine. A MEDLINE search in October 2004 found 6803 papers published on the topic. There are editorials, commentaries, reviews, case reports, accounts of technical innovation, as well as accounts of experiments and assessments. Although much (but not all) of this material is scholarly in character, only a limited number of studies could be regarded as evaluation. Evaluation implies a description or assessment with a view to answering a question or a set of questions. It is research, but research that aims to contribute to the making of a decision. The evaluation of telemedicine involves attempts to answer a wide range of questions involved in making decisions about safety, about practicality and about utility. Roughly speaking, if we wish to provide a telemedicine service we should first establish that it is safe, next that it is practical and finally that it is worthwhile. In evaluating telemedicine we focus on the systems, then on the service and finally on the health care that is provided.

Consider the following example. At a busy hospital there is a long waiting list for appointments to see dermatologists. It is therefore important that patients requiring urgent appointments are correctly identified, since a few skin conditions can be rapidly fatal. The only information available to the physician allocating appointments is that contained in the referral letter. Could a low-cost store-and-forward telemedicine service be used to provide the physician with an image of the patient's problem? How might we evaluate such a service? First, we would want to establish that the service is safe. We would want to be sure that the equipment we are using provides images of a sufficient quality to allow the doctors to assess the urgency with which an appointment is required. This means evaluating the camera and the link used to transmit the data, as well as the equipment used to view the images. It also means establishing what training is required for staff to be competent in using the system and what procedures must be followed to guarantee an appropriate level of care. The evaluations that are done in answering these questions take the form of laboratory-style experiments. They are performed in (relatively) controlled conditions and if they do involve real patients, the patients will probably be receiving the telemedicine consultation in addition to a conventional consultation.

Once it is established that a potential application is safe, it is then appropriate to ascertain whether it is feasible. Can we organize the service? Can the appropriate equipment be provided where it is needed? Are there people available who are competent to take the images and others capable of interpreting them? Can the required procedures be followed in practice? Are there additional financial or legal complications for the individuals and institutions involved? The evaluation that is done in answering these questions is an intermediate step between a laboratory study and a full trial, and takes the form of a pilot study or a small-scale trial.

When we know that the system and procedures are safe and that the proposed study is feasible, it remains to establish that the service can achieve worthwhile results. Is the service going to improve the quality of care that patients receive? Will it improve their health status? Is it cost-effective? In contrast to questions of safety, answering questions of effectiveness normally involves collecting data in the field; the service must first be implemented and data are then collected about the consequences of its implementation. In order to assess the effect of the telemedicine service, data for a comparison must also be collected, describing what happens, or what happened, in the absence of the service. Where such data are collected we say that the study is 'controlled'. Ideally, we wish to compare what happens where telemedicine is used (the intervention condition) with what happens when it is not used (the control condition) in the knowledge that the only difference between the conditions is the use of telemedicine. To be certain of this, the best thing to do is to assign patients (or consultations or doctors or hospitals or whatever the unit of study is) randomly to either the intervention or the control condition. Randomized controlled trials provide the most secure basis for valid causal inferences about the effects of medical interventions. It is difficult, but perfectly possible, to set up randomized controlled trials of telemedicine and a number of them have been reported. These have looked at a variety of telemedicine applications, such as the remote management of hypertension,[1] neurological outpatient appointments,[2] replacing general practitioner (GP) referral to hospital outpatient appointments,[3] teledermatology,[4] telepyschiatry[5] – see Table 8.1.

Where a number of well designed, robust studies have been carried out in the same field, addressing the same, similar or related questions, it is possible to carry out a systematic review to assess the overall quality of the evidence and draw a broad conclusion. The concept of a systematic review comes from the evidence-based medicine movement. The idea behind evidence-based medicine is that if patients are to reap the benefits of new research, clinicians must actively look for clinical evidence when making decisions about diagnosis and management. Advocates of evidence-based medicine around the world collaborate on identifying, collating and appraising all the available research on each of hundreds of specific questions, and publishing, for each, a systematic review, the results of which provide clinicians with a necessary short-cut to evidence-based practice. There have been in recent years a number of systematic reviews of telemedicine, some addressing particular outcomes (impact on clinical decision-

Table 8.1 Examples of randomized controlled trials of telemedicine

Author	Application	Intervention	Control	Outcomes measured	Conclusion
Friedman (1996)[1]	Monitoring hypertension in patients receiving therapy	Computer-based interactive telephone system for advice and counselling	Patients randomly assigned to normal care or to normal care plus intervention	Change in medication adherence; change in blood pressure	Improved medication adherence among non-adherents; improved blood pressure
Chua (2002)[2]	Neurological outpatient referrals	Assessment of new neurological outpatients at a district general hospital	Patients seen by neurologist randomly assigned to face-to-face assessment or telemedicine, also compared with a cohort seen face-to-face by GPs	Investigations ordered and disposal method (discharged, followed up as an outpatient, admitted)	Patients seen face to face by GPs received significantly more investigations and follow-up than other cohorts
Wallace (2002)[3]	Outpatient referrals in various clinical specialties	Replacing outpatient referrals with a videoconference between patient, GP and consultant	Patients randomly assigned to outpatient appointment or to videoconference	Patient satisfaction, subsequent health status, costs of treatments and investigations	Significant differences across different specialties. Overall patient satisfaction increased, but so did costs. Increased use of follow-up appointments
Collins (2004)[4]	Store-and-forward dermatology	GPs take still images of patients' lesions and send them, with clinical details, to a specialist	Patients randomly assigned to teledermatology or to outpatient appointment with a dermatologist	GP satisfaction	Significantly lower levels of satisfaction than indicated in other studies
Ruskin (2004)[5]	Treatment for depression	Psychiatric treatment delivered via video-conferencing over six months: psychoeducation, and brief supportive counselling	Depressed veterans referred for outpatient treatment randomly assigned to telepsychiatry or in-person treatment	Treatment outcomes, patient satisfaction and health-care costs	Comparable clinical outcomes and levels of patient satisfaction for equivalent level health-care cost

making,[6] on clinical outcomes,[7,8] patient satisfaction[9,10] and cost-effectiveness[8,11]), others addressing particular forms of telemedicine (electronic communication with patients,[12] videoconferencing in telepsychiatry[13]).

Systematic reviews, however, tend to focus on randomized controlled trials, and it is expensive and time-consuming to conduct such experiments. In some settings it is difficult, for ethical, administrative or scientific reasons, to organize the random assignment of patients to different conditions and so doctors, clinics, hospitals or even health authorities must be used as the unit of randomization. Such designs inevitably increase the number of observations required. The resources available for telemedicine research mean that only a limited number of randomized trials can be attempted. The best possible use must also be made of other forms of evaluation, including laboratory experiments and pilot studies.

Establishing the safety of telemedicine

The purpose of most safety studies in telemedicine is to show either that:

- the information of interest can be presented in a form using telemedicine that does not disadvantage its interpretation, compared with conventional methods of display;

or that:

- the overall process of management by telemedicine does not disadvantage the patient compared with care delivered by conventional means.

To this end, most laboratory studies of telemedicine have a common structure, and consist of the following steps:

(1) *Selection of cases.* Cases can be selected retrospectively in an image-based discipline (such as radiology) or prospectively. This might involve selecting cases to ensure the inclusion of a challenging set of conditions, or they might be unselected to ensure a natural mix of the easy and the difficult.
(2) *Interpretation.* Selected cases are interpreted in both a control and a telemedicine condition. Ideally, the same observers and the same cases will be used in both conditions. Learning effects are then counteracted by holding sessions some weeks apart, varying the order in which observers encounter the conditions and randomizing the presentation of cases.
(3) *Gold standard.* Some way of assessing the accuracy of the interpretations, by comparing them with a reference or 'gold standard', must also be found. Ideally, this would mean identifying a definitive test and applying this to each of the cases. This is rarely possible in practice and gold standards are either not obtained at all, or the consensus view of a set of experts is considered to be the true interpretation.

(4) *Statistical analyses.* Finally, the conclusions of interpreters in both conditions are compared with the gold standard and indices of comparative accuracy are calculated. The aim in these studies is to show that telemedicine is safe. The statistical test therefore is generally an attempt to fail to demonstrate a difference in accuracy (if a gold standard has been obtained) or an attempt to show a high level of agreement between observers in the two conditions (if a gold standard has not been obtained). Differences in accuracy are normally determined using ROC (receiver operating characteristic) analyses, whereas the statistic commonly used in measures of agreement is Cohen's kappa. Bland and Altman have suggested that the agreement between sets of measurements can best be assessed by plotting the difference between measurements against their mean. The standard deviation of differences between measurements made by two methods is a good indicator of the comparability of the methods.[14]

The issues surrounding patient safety include some of the most researched areas of telemedicine and some of these studies are extremely thorough. However, there are many difficulties in such studies and it is worth noting common problems. One frequent difficulty is that of extraneous differences between the control and intervention conditions. Telemedicine will generally require the use of unfamiliar equipment. It may also involve using equipment which has been temporarily installed in a location for another purpose. In such cases the comparison between the two conditions may not be a fair one.

A more fundamental problem concerns the assessment of results from safety studies. Studies have shown that radiologists can detect subtle lesions better using conventional film than using digital monitors. However, studies have also shown that very few abnormalities are missed when telemedicine is used to transmit unselected X-rays. For example, Gale *et al.*[15] found that major discrepancies between telemedicine interpretations and conventional film occurred in 1.5% of cases, compared with an inter-observer disagreement rate of 0.96% between radiologists interpreting conventional radiographic studies. Is this acceptable? If there is a clear advantage to be gained from the transmission of digital images, then the effect of the loss of information may be outweighed by the benefits. Determining this means moving from an assessment of safety to an evaluation of clinical benefits. If, for example, telemedicine is proposed as a means of providing consultant dermatology expertise in GP clinics, then consultants using the system must produce significantly more accurate results than those obtained by primary-care physicians in the absence of the system. How good are GPs at diagnosing dermatological problems? Basarab *et al.*[16] studied referrals by GPs to a dermatology clinic and found that only 47% of referral letters contained the correct diagnosis. It may therefore be that teledermatology could be valuable in primary care, even if the results for agreement between dermatologists seeing patients this way and also face to face are not perfect.

A telemedicine system must support the capture, transmission and display of medical information. If we are fully to understand how the safety of a diagnostic telemedicine application can be maximized, it is necessary to explore the effect of each of these three steps on the diagnostic performance of clinicians. In addition, there are issues about the ergonomics and usability of the systems employed. These different areas are considered below.

Information capture

The safety of an image capture device should be established in relation to the requirements of the intended application. For the purposes of some applications, such as teleconsultation, for which no standards have yet been defined, assessing the effect of the image capture stage is likely to involve experiments with different image capture devices to determine which is the most successful in a restricted number of actual teleconsultations. For other applications, however, a more defined course is necessary and any device will need to be assessed against known criteria for spatial and dynamic resolution. In the case of colour images the fidelity of the colour measurement is also an issue, as is the temporal resolution of live video images. Sadly, for most applications we know very little about these requirements. Some work has been done on the spatial and dynamic resolution required in radiology and pathology.[17-19] In dermatology Loane et al.[20] have shown improved accuracy in dermatological diagnosis using a camera with better colour resolution.

The susceptibility of the image capture device to variations in ambient conditions is also an issue. Vidmar[21] has described two experiences of forming an incorrect impression from images of skin lesions where additional views or improved lighting would have allowed an accurate diagnosis. Another important question concerns the skills required to capture appropriate images. Teleradiology services which seek to allow tertiary specialists to interpret images taken in other centres may be weakened by the absence of specialist nurses and radiographers to assist in the image capture process. Many studies of telepathology have used pathologists to capture the images, and yet a common source of error in such studies is that the wrong part of the slide was imaged: Halliday et al.[22] found a diagnostic error rate attributable specifically to this problem of 6.3%. If an expert pathologist is required to identify the appropriate image to transmit, there may be little additional value in a system for transmitting images to expert pathologists.

Information transmission

Determining the appropriate network connection for a telemedicine application is largely a matter of calculating the bandwidth required, although the reliability of the connection may be an issue in some applications. The requirements of live interactive video and of store-and-forward telemedicine are clearly different. The quantity of information to be transmitted depends on the size and resolution of the images, the number of images contained in a study and the extent to which the data can be compressed. Most videoconferencing applications transmit only the information required to update the image between successive frames and are able to transmit better video pictures if the movement between frames is minimized.

Zarate et al.[23] have compared the reliability of observers' assessments of schizophrenic patients at different bandwidths and found more reliable assessments at higher bandwidths (128 versus 384 kbit/s). Chan et al.[24] compared ISDN (128 and 384 kbit/s) to IP (768 kbit/s) and found the latter acceptable for the transmission of fetal ultrasound images.

The required bandwidth for a store-and-forward application is a function of the number of cases to be sent, the size and the number of images in a case, the extent to which data can be compressed, the case mix, the required turnaround and expectations of peak use.

Information display

One of the most thoroughly researched questions in telemedicine is that of the monitor characteristics required for the display of digital radiographs.[25] The performance of digital systems is now considered to be satisfactory for almost all applications of X-ray radiology, with the possible exception of mammography – where the results of definitive trials are still awaited. It is worth noting that many radiologists prefer to interpret images on film and it is standard practice in many hospitals to print digital images onto film for radiologists to interpret. The advantages of film are in part to do with familiarity, but there are others: it is easy to view a large number of films displayed simultaneously on a light box, to move films around and place them side by side. Light boxes are often more thoughtfully positioned than computer display terminals.

There are a number of parameters defining the quality of the display, the most obvious being the number of pixels and the number of bits per pixel that the screen can display. The spatial resolution of a displayed image, however, is a function not just of the size of the screen matrix but also of the precision of the phosphor display. Different devices have different characteristics and the display of subtle changes in colour may be particularly susceptible to such variations. The power of the display monitor is also a factor in determining the perceptibility of contrast. Some studies have found that the contrast resolution of a display is often substantially less in practice than that specified by the manufacturer.[26] In telemedicine applications based on videoconferencing, the picture rate is a factor and so too is the quality of sound.

Ergonomics

The usability of both the capture and display software is important. Most display systems attempt to compensate for inadequate rendering of spatial and contrast resolution by allowing the user to scroll and zoom an image, and to adjust the display characteristics such as brightness and contrast. The interface provided for these tools, and for any other image-processing facilities, is a factor that affects the usability of the system.

Reviewing the evidence on safety

Hersh et al.[6] have published a systematic review of the evidence about telemedicine's impact on clinical decision making. Fifty-nine relevant studies were identified. They concluded that there was evidence that decisions made on the basis of telemedicine were comparable to those made face to face, but that this evidence was limited to a few clinical specialties and a limited number of decisions. There were well designed studies providing good evidence that telemedicine worked well in psychiatry and dermatology, for history taking and clinical examinations in general medicine and cardiology, and for certain areas of ophthalmology. They noted that the overall methodological quality of the studies reviewed was low, and that many studies had small sample sizes, that the same clinician often looked at cases in both conditions (with and without telemedicine) and that few researchers measured inter-observer agreement.

Establishing the practicality of telemedicine

There have been many pilot studies of telemedicine and a great many articles have been published as accounts of pilot studies. Most of these studies have been carried out as demonstrations, to show that a proposed application can be implemented in a chosen setting.

Some accounts of pilot studies provide illuminating comments on decisions taken or difficulties encountered. For example, Harrison et al.[27] wrote that it proved difficult to get all the required parties together to hold a realtime teleconsultation and their experience suggested a 'feasibility ceiling' of two to three teleconsultations per week for a general practitioner. Brecht et al.[28] described the first phase of a project to provide teleconsultations for the Texas prison service. Their goal of 100 scheduled teleconsultations per week was not met because of difficulties in transporting patients to the telemedicine facility, an overall drop in referrals – due to a review of the referral process – and the cancellation of clinics due to a lack of available specialists.

These observations are useful, but in general the literature on telemedicine contains disappointingly little information about when telemedicine applications are or are not practical. One would like to be able to abstract from the experience gained in these pilot studies a set of principles about implementation and installation: principles which could then be applied in other studies and subjected to some form of empirical examination and possibly altered or refined. The installation and implementation of telemedicine may not be sufficiently distinctive to warrant such an analysis, but if it is not then one would expect to see methodologies for managing other kinds of computer projects being employed.

A number of investigators have used qualitative research, including the kinds of ethnographic studies developed in the social sciences, to study projects in which a telemedicine solution had been attempted but had failed to gain acceptance.[29] These investigations contribute to our understanding of the social and organizational barriers that must be overcome if telemedicine is to be applied successfully. For example, May et al.[30] carried out an ethnographic study of a telepsychiatry pilot and found that the health-care professionals, who had initially expected that the technology would improve the efficiency with which they worked, discovered that they were unable to establish the kind of emotional rapport with their patients that seemed to be an essential basis for a therapeutic relationship. (Notwithstanding this, telepsychiatry is practised routinely in many parts of the world.)

Telemedicine projects are not guaranteed to succeed. Some telemedicine services have failed to meet a real need, failed to take account of the constraints imposed by the local organization of health care or failed to consider the practices of the relevant staff. It is also true that apparent success in the pilot phase of a project – which will largely involve enthusiasts for the technology – is not an absolute guarantee of real success later on.

Establishing the effectiveness of telemedicine

In some applications telemedicine can be used to improve the efficiency of an existing service, for example in enhancing the communication at the primary–secondary care interface.[3] In others, telemedicine can be used to make an existing service available to a new community, for example allowing a specialist radiologist to interpret images taken at other centres.[31] It can also be used to provide a new kind of service, for example allowing pregnant women to have their blood pressure monitored at home.[32] In each of these cases, the introduction of telemedicine represents an intervention at a different level in the organization of health care and it follows that in each case the outcomes that must be assessed in any evaluation will be different. If telemedicine is introduced as a refinement of the existing process of health care, it may be sufficient to measure variables that, essentially, provide information about the process. Where telemedicine is used to provide a new or different kind of service, it is necessary to concentrate on measures of outcome rather than process. In any case, it is inevitably outcomes that we are interested in and it will always be preferable to measure outcomes where possible.

The choice of outcome measure depends in part on the aim with which the telemedicine service was set up. If the original motivation was to avoid patient transfers, any evaluation of the service must measure the subsequent change in the number of transfers. Since the service may have an effect on a number of other variables, these should also be assessed, to allow an overall evaluation of the costs and benefits of the service. Outcome measures found in evaluations of telemedicine services can be divided into three categories: measures of user satisfaction, measures of medical outcome and financial measures.

User satisfaction
The attitudes of patients to the use of telemedicine have been measured by many authors, with most reporting high levels of satisfaction and a willingness to use telemedicine in the future.[9,10] The measures of satisfaction used generally relate to how patients rate the process of consultation and how effective they perceive the

consultation to have been. Most researchers therefore measure patient ratings of teleconsultation as a means of communication, asking specifically about whether patients could see and hear everything, and whether or not they felt they could express themselves as fully as they could have in a normal consultation. Patients are usually questioned about how the process of consultation made them feel and whether or not issues of privacy or confidentiality concerned them.

Researchers, assessing patients' perceptions of the effectiveness of a consultation, usually ask if patients have confidence in teleconsultation as a means of managing their problems. Researchers also tend to ask patients whether teleconsultations are as good as conventional care. In assessing the value of such judgements, however, it should be remembered that patients' perceptions of conventional medicine might not be very accurate. Many patients will not be able to judge the relative accuracy of telemedicine and conventional medicine, since few will be aware of the probability of receiving a misdiagnosis from a conventional consultation. (In fact, remarkably little information on this point exists in the literature.) Also, patients might be expected to prefer telemedicine to conventional medicine if they perceive that it offers them an improved service. This is a major problem because patients may receive better treatment as a result of their participation in a research trial and this can engender a false degree of satisfaction with telemedicine. It is often said that telemedicine will improve patients' access to specialist expertise. However, in most studies using telemedicine to connect patients to hospital consultants, it is the participation in a research study that allows patients to skip the waiting list associated with a conventional appointment.

Other authors have also assessed the attitudes of clinicians. The measures of satisfaction used in these studies do have areas which are common to those questions asked of patients, such as measures of process and effectiveness. It is, however, common to question clinicians specifically about organizational issues, for example how easy it was to coordinate the teleconsultation, how easy it was to make contact with the specialist, and how easy it was to use the equipment.

Whitten et al.[33] surveyed physicians' attitudes to a telemedicine service. All were aware of telemedicine and positive about its advantages, but only nine (32%) had used it. Three main reasons were given for the lack of use: the training was inadequate, the service did not fit existing referral patterns and there were organizational problems. Shile et al.[34] found that a telemedicine link between an emergency room and a radiology department was little used. In all, 19% of films were never digitized and it was possible for clinicians to obtain the information they required just as quickly through conventional channels. Mitchell et al.[35] surveyed staff involved in the installation of a videoconferencing system connecting four renal dialysis centres. The most frequently mentioned problems were difficulty in moving the equipment, absence of privacy and awkward lighting. These problems were all mentioned more frequently than ones such as image quality, which are the subject of most telemedicine research. Franken et al.[36] surveyed the staff of a community hospital where radiological services were provided by: (1) teleradiology; (2) a radiologist visiting two or three times a week; (3) a radiologist in daily attendance; or (4) a radiologist being present during working hours. No difference was found between the services in terms of diagnostic accuracy. The telemedicine service, however, received a negative evaluation on all criteria other than courtesy.

Reviewing the evidence on patient satisfaction

There have been two systematic reviews of patient satisfaction. The first, by Williams et al.,[9] identified 93 studies across a range of specialties (the best represented being telepsychiatry, multispecialty care, nursing and dermatology). The majority (88%) were of videoconferencing applications. Reported levels of satisfaction with telemedicine were consistently greater than 80%, and were frequently 100%. The reviewers, however, report significant methodological weaknesses in much of the research. One-third of the studies involved fewer than 20 patients and only 20% included a control group. Similar criticisms were made by Mair and Whitten,[10] following a review of 32 studies, often with small sample sizes, poor response rates and poorly specified recruitment criteria. Few studies defined what satisfaction meant. Nevertheless, the reviewers noted that patients generally found telemedicine acceptable and noted definite advantages, while occasionally expressing disquiet.

Medical outcomes

Studies of the safety of telemedicine generally attempt to show that there is no significant difference between conventional medicine and telemedicine, so that there is no negative effect on patient outcome from the use of telemedicine. Extrapolating from this, it is assumed that there will be a positive effect, in terms of quality of care, cost-effectiveness or improved accessibility. There have, however, been relatively few attempts to demonstrate that telemedicine actually improves patients' health, and even fewer successful attempts. Goh et al.[37] studied the use of telemedicine to transmit CT scans of neurosurgical patients. They compared 50 referrals made without teleradiology with 66 referrals made following teleradiology, and found a 21% reduction in unnecessary transfers and a significant reduction in adverse events during transfer (8% versus 32%).

Darkins et al.[38] investigated the effect of a videoconferencing facility on the management of patients at a minor treatment centre (i.e. a small-hospital emergency department staffed by nurse practitioners, not doctors). A standard videoconferencing system was used to connect the centre to a hospital accident and emergency department. The investigators noticed a marked change in referral practices following the introduction of the system. It seems likely that this was largely due to telemedicine. However, as the authors pointed out, the weakness of such before-and-after comparisons is that one cannot be certain that telemedicine was the cause of the observed effect. The centre had been open for only a year before the telemedicine system was introduced and it is likely that part of the effect was due to changes in patients' attitudes to the centre.

The surest basis for making judgements of cause and effect is a randomized controlled trial. Telemonitoring has been the subject of such a trial in the context of a system to support patients with hypertension.[1] Users measured their blood pressure at home and received advice and counselling from a computer system accessed via an ordinary touch-tone telephone. The mean antihypertensive medication adherence improved by 18% for the system users and 12% for controls. Mean diastolic blood pressure, measured at the patients' home in both the study and control condition, decreased by 5.2 mmHg (660 Pa) in users and 0.8 mmHg (106 Pa) in controls.

Reviewing the evidence on clinical outcomes

Hersh *et al.*[7] carried out a systematic review of the evidence on the impact of telemedicine on clinical outcomes and concluded that there was only a limited amount of good evidence of favourable outcomes. They identified 25 studies meeting their inclusion criteria. The best evidence came from applications designed to deliver care in patients' homes, with favourable outcomes found for patients with chronic disease, AIDS and Alzheimer's disease. The evidence from trials of the home monitoring of diabetes is mixed, with one large well designed trial of a system for paediatric patients showing no difference between the control and intervention groups. Two large adult studies have similarly proved negative, while others have demonstrated a benefit. Relatively few trials of hospital-based outpatient or inpatient telemedicine applications have looked at clinical outcomes. In addition to the teleradiology applications mentioned above, beneficial effects have been shown by studies of telemedicine in the emergency department, intensive care unit (ICU) and surgery. In a before–after study of the introduction of a telemedicine system to allow intensivists continuously to oversee patients in an ICU, there was a significant reduction in mortality, length of stay and complications.[39]

Financial measures

The systematic review of assessments of telemedicine by Roine *et al.*[8] reported that there were few studies demonstrating cost benefit from the introduction of a telemedicine service. This may, in part, be explained by the fact that calculating the true effects of telemedicine on a health-care delivery system can be extremely difficult. The studies that have been performed have instead tended to concentrate on the short-term implications of an easily defined part of the overall process, rarely attempting to take a societal view of the effect of such interventions. McIntosh and Cairns[40] described areas that might be considered in such an approach.

Most of the published economic evaluations of telemedicine have, however, been based on more straightforward calculations. In highly constrained settings, this can be quite appropriate. Studies of the cost-effectiveness of telemedicine in these situations have found that savings are possible. Brunicardi[41] found that the mean cost of a medical consultation in the Ohio prison system was $263, and that this dropped to $255 using telemedicine. Increased use of telemedicine would further reduce the unit cost per consultation.

Studies conducted in the community have shown that telemedicine is a viable financial alternative. For example, Mahmud and Lenz[42] described a telemonitoring project in which two-way videophones, blood pressure and pulse monitors, electronic stethoscopes and emergency response systems were installed in patients' homes. In seven out of 12 patients, there was a reduction in the frequency of home nursing visits. The cost of a video nursing visit worked out at US$15 against US$90 for a home visit. Bergmo[43] compared the costs of patient travel, visiting specialists and teleconsultations for an otorhinolaryngology service in Norway. Teleconsultation was found to be cost-effective for workloads between 56 and 325 patients a year. Two UK trials have looked at the cost-effectiveness of videoconferencing between primary and secondary care as an alternative to outpatient appointments. One large randomized controlled trial that used telemedicine to replace GP referrals across a range of specialties found some savings in, for example, the number of tests ordered, but these were generally low-cost tests and, overall, the intervention substantially increased costs.[44] A similar study focusing on teledermatology found that the high fixed costs associated with telemedicine meant that the teledermatology service was more expensive, but that an increased patient throughput could have led to reduced societal costs, especially for patients in rural areas.[45]

Two studies have considered the cost-effectiveness of teleradiology. Halvorsen and Kristiansen[46] considered a random sample of the radiological examinations required by a GP centre in Norway. They estimated the costs under three models, one in which all examinations were performed at the nearest hospital (140 km away), one in which GPs interpreted some examinations taken locally and one in which teleradiology was used to avoid unnecessary hospital referrals. Of the 553 referrals analysed, teleradiology was considered an option for 389 (the others required scans not supported by the proposed teleradiology service, or were concurrently referred for other services). The costs of the different options were not very different. Interestingly, this study is sometimes cited as if it provided support for telemedicine even though the authors stated that they included favourable estimates of the costs of teleradiology, optimum utilization was assumed and estimates of depreciation and maintenance were chosen from the lower end of the scale. Bergmo[47] considered the costs of the teleradiology service provided by the University Hospital of Tromsø to the Military Hospital, two and a half hours' drive away. Taking into account the fixed and variable costs of a teleradiology and a conventional radiology service, the author concluded that the service was cost-effective for workloads above 1576 patients per annum (Figure 8.1). The service was described as performing 8000 examinations per year.

Neither of these studies was a field trial. In both, the costs of providing the service in one way were known and compared with costs that might have been incurred had the service been provided the other way. Estimating such costs is always a difficult business, and particularly so in telemedicine, where the costs per case are very dependent on the use made of the service, something that can be very hard to predict.

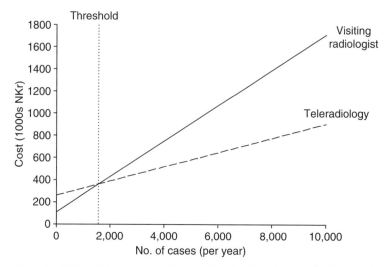

Figure 8.1 Costs of teleradiology and a visiting radiologist (from Bergmo[47]). The threshold at which teleradiology becomes cheaper than a visiting radiologist occurs at 1576 cases per year

One difficulty with these studies is that a comparison between telemedicine and current practice may suggest that telemedicine is cost-effective even though there is a much cheaper alternative. Not all transactions between patient and doctor require face-to-face contact and it would seem unlikely that all such transactions require high-resolution, high-bandwidth and high-fidelity interactive television.

Reviewing the evidence on cost-effectiveness

Whitten *et al.*[11] carried out a systematic review of studies of the cost-effectiveness of telemedicine. They identified 612 articles but found actual cost–benefit data only in 55, of which 20 concluded that telemedicine saved money. However, the reviewers found that only 24 of the 55 articles met their quality criteria and they argue that none adequately addressed the question of whether telemedicine provides value for money. For example, no studies used a cost–utility approach and none adequately addressed the question of the potential benefits that could accrue from economies of scale if telemedicine was more widely available. Most projects are too short in duration to allow reliable estimates to be made of what a fully established service would cost. The reviewers conclude that the paucity of research, the low technical quality, poor design and inappropriate analysis mean that no useful conclusions can be drawn about the cost-effectiveness of telemedicine.

Conclusion

The term 'telemedicine' exists because computer-derived images transmitted over digital networks have made us think about how medicine might be practised at a distance. But even if it is technology that has raised the question, it does not follow that technology is, necessarily, the solution. One of the difficulties is that the vendors of relatively expensive telemedicine systems and services disseminate much of the information on the topic. We have to focus not on the glamorous technology but on the underlying issue of how the participants in health care (patients, GPs, specialists) can communicate more effectively, using the range of technological options open to them. A systematic review of electronic communication with patients found many successful examples of innovative uses of relatively low-technology telephone services in counselling, reminders, follow-up and other applications.[12]

Ensuring that the most appropriate technology is used in the most effective way should be the primary aim of telemedicine research. This means first establishing the requirements of the proposed application through careful studies of the effect of various parameters on the capture, transmission and display of information and then moving to an assessment of the impact of the service following a suitable pilot. It will never be possible to study all the variables involved in a complex intervention like telemedicine. The resources available for research are limited and the pace of technical and organizational change limits the value of exhaustive study. As in any other research programme, it is essential to take as much as possible from what has already been learnt and to focus on the issues that remain to be explored.

Perhaps the most interesting question about telemedicine concerns the likely effect of the technology on referral patterns. Some authors have suggested that a principal benefit of telemedicine will be to reduce waiting times. Consider the effects that telemedicine could have on the use made of consultant time. It could result in an overall decrease in the number of appointments, because the interactions with GPs facilitated by the system mean that GPs are able to manage more patients without requiring referrals. Dermatologists have argued that improvements in GP training and better support for community-based care would drastically reduce the demand for consultant appointments. Another effect, however, might produce the opposite result. Some research suggests that many patients who should be referred are not referred, and that more knowledgeable GPs have higher referral rates.[48] It is also possible that the availability of telemedicine will encourage more referrals. Telemedicine might actually have the effect of increasing the pressure on consultant time. Furthermore, realtime telemedicine consultations seem to take longer than conventional ones and are difficult to schedule.[39] At the moment, it is simply not possible to say if the benefits will outweigh the costs.

A huge amount has been published about telemedicine. Recent systematic reviews have highlighted the poor quality of much of this work. However, as the field matures, the number of well designed, robust evaluations is increasing. There is now sufficient evidence for us to be confident that telemedicine is a safe alternative to conventional care in a variety of situations, and for a number of clinical conditions. Reliable evidence that it is a practical and cost-effective alternative is, at the time of writing, harder to find.

References

1   Friedman RH, Kazis LE, Jette A, *et al*. A telecommunications system for monitoring and counseling patients with hypertension. *Am J Hypertens* 1996;**9**:285–92

2   Chua R, Craig J, Esmonde T, Wootton R, Patterson V. Putting a randomized controlled trial in the context of everyday practice. *J Telemed Telecare* 2002;**8**:270–3

3   Wallace P, Haines A, Harrison R, *et al*. Joint teleconsultations (virtual outreach) versus standard outpatient appointments for patients referred by their general practitioner for a specialist opinion: a randomised trial. *Lancet* 2002;**359**:1961–8

4   Collins K, Bowns I, Walters S. General practitioners' perceptions of asynchronous telemedicine in a randomized controlled trial of teledermatology. *J Telemed Telecare* 2004;**10**:94–8

5   Ruskin PE, Silver-Aylaian M, Kling MA, *et al*. Treatment outcomes in depression: comparison of remote treatment through telepsychiatry to in-person treatment. *Am J Psychiatry* 2004;**161**:1471–6

6   Hersh W, Helfand M, Wallace J, *et al*. A systematic review of the efficacy of telemedicine for making diagnostic and management decisions. *J Telemed Telecare* 2002;**8**:197–209

7   Hersh WR, Helfand M, Wallace J, *et al*. Clinical outcomes resulting from telemedicine interventions: a systematic review. *BMC Med Inform Decis Mak* 2001;**1**:5

8   Roine R, Ohinmaa A, Hailey D. Assessing telemedicine: a systematic review of the literature. *CMAJ* 2001;**165**:765–71

9   Williams TL, May CR, Esmail A. Limitations of patient satisfaction studies in telehealthcare: a systematic review of the literature. *Telemed J E Health* 2002;**7**:293–316

10   Mair F, Whitten P. Systematic review of studies of patient satisfaction with telemedicine. *BMJ* 2000;**320**:1517–20

11   Whitten PS, Mair FS, Haycox A, May CR, Williams TL, Hellmich S. Systematic review of cost effectiveness studies of telemedicine interventions. *BMJ* 2002;**324**:1434–7

12   Balas EA, Jaffrey F, Kuperman GJ, *et al*. Electronic communication with patients. Evaluation of distance medicine technology. *JAMA* 1997;**278**:152–9

13   Pesamaa L, Ebeling H, Kuusimaki ML, Winblad I, Isohanni M, Moilanen I. Videoconferencing in child and adolescent telepsychiatry: a systematic review of the literature. *J Telemed Telecare* 2004;**10**:187–92

14   Bland M, Altman D. Statistical methods for assessing agreement between two methods of clinical measurement. *Lancet* 1986;**1**:307–10

15   Gale ME, Vincent ME, Robbins AH. Teleradiology for remote diagnosis: a prospective multi-year evaluation. *J Digit Imaging* 1997;**10**:47–50

16   Basarab T, Munn SE, Jones RR. Diagnostic accuracy and appropriateness of general practitioner referrals to a dermatology out-patient clinic. *Br J Dermatol* 1996;**135**:70–3

17   American College of Radiology. *Standard for Teleradiology*. American College of Radiology, 2003. See http://www.acr.org/s_acr/index.asp (last checked 13 January 2005)

18   Benger J, Lock A, Cook J, Kendall J. The effect of resolution, compression, colour depth and display modality on the accuracy of accident and emergency telemedicine. *J Telemed Telecare* 2001;**7** (Suppl. 1):6–7

19   Williams BH, Hong IS, Mullick FG, Butler DR, Herring RF, O'Leary TJ. Image quality issues in a static image-based telepathology consultation practice. *Hum Pathol* 2003;**34**:1228–34

20   Loane MA, Gore HE, Corbett R, *et al*. Effect of camera performance on diagnostic accuracy: preliminary results from the Northern Ireland arms of the UK Multicentre Teledermatology Trial. *J Telemed Telecare* 1997;**3**:83–8

21   Vidmar DA. Plea for standardization in dermatology: a worm's eye view. *Telemed J* 1997;**3**:173–8

22   Halliday BE, Bhattacharyya AK, Graham AR, *et al*. Diagnostic accuracy of an international static-imaging telepathology consultation service. *Hum Pathol* 1997;**28**:17–21

23   Zarate CA, Weinstock L, Cukor P, *et al*. Applicability of telemedicine for assessing patients with schizophrenia: acceptance and reliability. *J Clin Psychiatry* 1997;**58**:22–5

24   Chan FY, Taylor A, Soong B, *et al*. Randomized comparison of the quality of realtime fetal ultrasound images transmitted by ISDN and by IP videoconferencing. *J Telemed Telecare* 2002;**8**:91–6

25   Krupinski E. Practical applications of perceptual research. In: Beutel J, Kundel H, Van Metter R, eds. *Handbook of Medical Imaging. Vol 1: Physics and Psychophysics*. Bellingham: SPIE Press, 2000

26   Lo SC, Gaskill JW, Mun SK, Krasner BH. Contrast information of digital imaging in laser film digitizer and display monitor. *J Digit Imaging* 1990;**3**:119–23

27   Harrison R, Clayton W, Wallace P. Can telemedicine be used to improve communication between primary and secondary care? *BMJ* 1996;**313**:1377–81

28   Brecht RM, Gray CL, Peterson C, Youngblood B. The University of Texas Medical Branch–Texas Department of Criminal Justice Telemedicine Project: findings from the first year of operation. *Telemed J* 1996;**2**:23–35

29   May C, Harrison R, Finch T, MacFarlane A, Mair F, Wallace P. Understanding the normalization of telemedicine services through qualitative evaluation. *J Am Med Inform Assoc* 2003;**10**:596–604

30   May C, Gask L, Atkinson T, Ellis N, Mair F, Esmail A. Resisting and promoting new technologies in clinical practice: the case of telepsychiatry. *Soc Sci Med* 2001;**52**:1889–901

31   Franken Jr EA, Berbaum KS, Brandser EA, D'Alessandro MP, Schweiger GD, Smith WL. Pediatric radiology at a rural hospital: value of teleradiology and subspecialty consultation. *Am J Roentgenol* 1997;**168**:1349–52

32   Naef III RW, Perry Jr KG, Magann EF, McLaughlin BN, Chauhan SP, Morrison JC. Home blood pressure monitoring for pregnant patients with hypertension. *J Perinatol* 1998;**18**:226–9

33   Whitten P, Franken EA. Telemedicine for patient consultation: factors affecting use by rural primary care physcians in Kansas. *J Telemed Telecare* 1995;**1**:139–44

34   Shile PE, Kundel HL, Seshadri SB, *et al.* Factors affecting the electronic communication of radiological information to an intensive-care unit. *J Telemed Telecare* 1996;**2**:199–204

35   Mitchell BR, Mitchell JG, Disney AP. User adoption issues in renal telemedicine. *J Telemed Telecare* 1996;**2**:81–6

36   Franken Jr EA, Whitten P, Smith WL. Teleradiology services for a rural hospital: a case study. *J Telemed Telecare* 1996;**2**:155–60

37   Goh KY, Lam CK, Poon WS. The impact of teleradiology on the inter-hospital transfer of neurosurgical patients. *Br J Neurosurg* 1997;**11**:52–6

38   Darkins A, Dearden CH, Rocke LG, Martin JB, Sibson L, Wootton R. An evaluation of telemedical support for a minor treatment centre. *J Telemed Telecare* 1996;**2**:93–9

39   Rosenfeld BA, Dorman T, Breslow MJ, *et al.* Intensive care unit telemedicine: alternate paradigm for providing continuous intensivist care. *Crit Care Med* 2000;**28**:3925–31

40   McIntosh E, Cairns J. A framework for the economic evaluation of telemedicine. *J Telemed Telecare* 1997;**3**:132–9

41   Brunicardi BO. Financial analysis of savings from telemedicine in Ohio's prison system. *Telemed J* 1998;**4**:49–54

42   Mahmud K, Lenz L. The personal telemedicine system. A new tool for the delivery of health care. *J Telemed Telecare* 1995;**1**:173–7

43   Bergmo TS. An economic analysis of teleconsultation in otorhinolaryngology. *J Telemed Telecare* 1997;**3**:194–9

44   Jacklin PB, Roberts JA, Wallace P, *et al.* Virtual outreach: economic evaluation of joint teleconsultations for patients referred by their general practitioner for a specialist opinion. *BMJ* 2003;**327**:84

45   Loane MA, Bloomer SE, Corbett R, *et al.* A randomized controlled trial assessing the health economics of realtime teledermatology compared with conventional care: an urban versus rural perspective. *J Telemed Telecare* 2001;**7**:108–18

46   Halvorsen PA, Kristiansen IS. Radiology services for remote communities. *BMJ* 1996;**312**:1333–1336

47   Bergmo TS. An economic analysis of teleradiology versus a visiting radiologist service. *J Telemed Telecare* 1996;**2**:136–42

48   Reynolds GA, Chitnis JG, Roland MO. General practitioner outpatient referrals: do good doctors refer more patients to hospital? *BMJ* 1991;**302**:1250–2

Further information

1   Bowling A. *Research Methods in Health.* Buckingham: Open University Press, 2002

2   Khan K, Kunz R, Kleijnen J, Antes G. *Systematic Reviews to Support Evidence-Based Medicine.* London: Royal Society of Medicine Press, 2004

3   HTA. *The NHS Health Technology Assessment Programme.* See http://www.ncchta.org/ (last checked 7 January 2005)

4   Friedman CP, Wyatt J. *Evaluation Methods in Medical Informatics.* New York: Springer-Verlag, 1997

▶9

How to do a telemedical consultation

James Ferguson

Introduction

What is a telemedical consultation? To consult is to seek information or advice from someone.[1] Therefore, a telemedical consultation is to seek medical information or advice from someone at a distance.[2] The consultation may be from patient to health-care professional or between health-care professionals. A teleconsultation may be required for reasons of distance. For example, a remote site with no health-care personnel (e.g. a fishing vessel) may be reliant on telecommunications to access health-care advice. A teleconsultation may also be required where access to expert advice is difficult. For example, in a busy specialist clinic, junior doctors or specialist nurses may undertake data collection and present information to the specialist for advice with no direct contact between the specialist and patient, despite their being in the same building.

Consultation by telephone, particularly in primary care, is accepted as an integral part of routine practice. However, teleconsultation techniques are not taught routinely. This has led to teleconsultation being regarded with suspicion as an inferior substitute for person-to-person contact, despite good evidence to the contrary in terms of safety and patient satisfaction.[3]

Global shortages of medical staff have driven changes in medical care delivery to make the best use of available resources. Health-care professionals often migrate to larger conurbations, making the situation worse in remote and rural environments. The European Working Time Directive limiting hours of work has further exacerbated the staff shortage, particularly in the areas of out-of-hours care and specialist advice.[4] Teleconsultation to deliver routine care may be considered only when a service is under pressure and alternative solutions such as increasing the medical workforce are not possible.

Increased utilization of teleconsultations may help to alleviate staff shortages. For example, suitably trained pre-hospital practitioners (e.g. paramedics or nurses) may safely deliver unscheduled care, previously delivered primarily by doctors, with decision support from a medical practitioner via communications technology.[5]

Health-care professionals must become proficient at consulting with patients and other health-care professionals at a distance and with the technology available to facilitate this. Teleconsultation should therefore become an integral part of health-care training.

Principles of consultation

To elaborate on the definition given above, a consultation is an exchange of data to solve a problem.[6] The level of complexity varies dramatically. It may be a simple exchange of information, such as a patient calling a nurse advice line to determine the opening times of local pharmacies. At its most complex, a consultation may involve sophisticated data exchange. For example, a consultation for chest pain may involve collection of extensive data such as past medical history, clinical findings and an electrocardiogram (ECG) before advice is given on treatment (Figure 9.1). The majority of diagnoses may be made on history alone. Therefore, a well focused discussion with a patient will reveal the majority of the relevant data. The role of non-verbal communication in medical consultation is significant, especially in general practice, where as many as 55% of patients present with symptoms unrelated to the main reason for seeking help.[6]

Examination is commonly taught and performed as a checklist of signs to be elicited and recorded. However, experienced clinicians will undertake focused clinical examination to confirm or rule out diagnoses suggested by the history. A full clinical examination is not necessary for *all* consultations. Clinical examination is an important part of consultation but should always be regarded as an adjunct to good history taking. Similarly, inexperienced clinicians frequently order investigations in a 'blanket-like' fashion to cover major

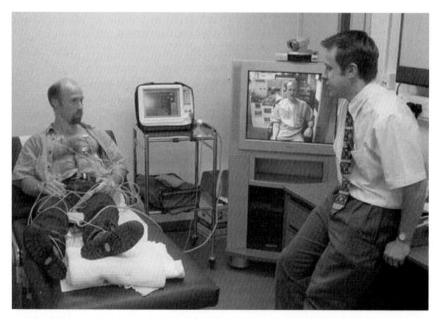

Figure 9.1 Videoconferencing combined with ECG telemetry for a patient with a suspected myocardial infarction

diagnoses, instead of focusing on those investigations where the result might alter the management of the patient.

It follows that data collection depends on the nature of the consultation. A general practice consultation for a repeat prescription may simply require a verbal review of the patient's progress. A psychological consultation may require discussion of symptoms, although body language may be a vital component of the data. A dermatology consultation requires a comprehensive medical history combined with visualizing the skin and examination. A cardiac consultation may require history, examination and investigation for a diagnosis to be made.

Clinicians who are considering the use of teleconsultation must reflect objectively on their role in, and data requirements from, a consultation. The clinician should identify the most discriminatory pieces of data required to make a diagnosis. Some data may be elicited only by direct contact with a patient (e.g. abdominal palpation, stressing knee ligaments, ECG). However, in the majority of cases, sufficient data to enable successful consultation may be collected directly by telemedicine or by a remote practitioner working as a proxy for the specialist.

Teleconsultation media

What techniques are available for teleconsultation? The communications medium will depend on the type of consultation. The consultation itself may occur directly between the patient and a health-care professional, or via a third party. Their interaction may be asynchronous or synchronous.

Asynchronous consultation

An asynchronous consultation involves data being sent for assessment by the consulting health-care professional at a later time. Prior to the development of electronic communications technology, doctors would write to specialists, describing their patient's symptoms and seeking advice. Even today, readers write to magazines describing their symptoms and the letter and the specialist's advice are published. These represent examples of simple asynchronous tele-consultation.

Asynchronous consultation is being increasingly used in routine health care. There are various Websites on the Internet where an individual may list symptoms and advice is offered. Unfortunately, lack of effective regulation of the Internet means that the quality of the advice is variable and only reliable sites should be recommended, e.g. the NHS24 online site (http://www.nhsdirect.nhs.uk/), but even for these evidence of long-term safety is lacking.

Initially, electronic mail (email) was used for administrative purposes but, increasingly, it is being used for clinical care as well. Questionnaires completed by the patient may be attached, as may clinical information such as pictures, ECG recordings and audio files. The effectiveness of email for teleconsultation has been well documented in dermatology,[7] general medicine[8] and neurology.[9]

The use of email in acute situations is increasing, for example transmission of ECG files from patients with acute chest pain. New inexpensive software to capture ECGs combined with the cost-effectiveness, robustness and familiarity of email make this a viable and acceptable option. Self-capture and transmission of ECG data by patients has recently been described.[10]

An advantage of asynchronous communication is that the two parties do not have to be present for the transfer of data. This is commonly referred to as 'store and forward' communication and lends itself to non-emergency conditions mainly. Its success relies on relevant data being supplied to the specialist by the patient or remote health-care professional. In routine practice, this is facilitated by the use of questionnaires developed by the advising health-care professional (e.g. a dermatologist), which focuses on data essential to make a diagnosis.

As with any type of teleconsultation, clear objectives and pre-planning results in increased effectiveness. Some 80–90% of dermatological conditions may be diagnosed via asynchronous consultation.[7]

Synchronous consultation

Synchronous teleconsultation occurs in realtime at a distance using communications technology. In general terms, increasingly complex medical conditions require more sophisticated teleconsultation media to allow effective delivery of care.

Consultation by telephone is used extensively. Frequently, this occurs directly between the patient and a health-care professional. Up to 70% of out-of-hours primary care contacts with general practitioners are dealt with by telephone advice alone. Telephone medical advice lines are proliferating in many countries and the National Health Service line in Britain, NHS24/Direct, represents the world's largest single teleconsultation service.[11]

Telephone advice is routinely sought between health-care professionals, such as clinical consultants advising general practitioners (GPs) or junior staff. The proliferation of mobile telephony, including the ability to send images and data files to portable wireless devices, has the potential to significantly improve access to specialist advice, particularly in emergency situations.[12]

Radio communications have been used to advise on medical situations since the development of radio. Radio communication is used in many settings, such as in providing advice to ships.[13] Duplex radio transmission resembles use of a telephone (i.e. both parties may talk at once) but requires a radio link of sufficient capacity. If capacity is limited, simplex contact may be used (only one person may talk at a time) and the participants in a teleconsultation must take account of this. Teleconsultation may be enhanced by a pro forma being completed by the remote carer. The answers may then be converted to alphanumeric data, which decreases transmission time and increases clarity in conditions of limited duration or poor-quality contact. The advisers decode the message and construct a reply.

Telemetry allows realtime transmission of physiological data from the patient to a health-care provider. This may include variables such as blood pressure, pulse rate and oxygen saturation. Transfer of realtime ECG data has been used to diagnose and rapidly treat myocardial infarction, as well as to monitor postoperative cardiac patients at home. Currently, the equipment is expensive, which limits use of the technique to specific situations where specialist medical advice is required.

None of the above examples involves the health-care professional seeing the patient. Videoconferencing allows direct visualization and dialogue with the patient, which more closely re-creates the traditional consultation environment. Transfer of visual data facilitates 'pattern recognition' and allows better rapport to be developed between the patient and the health-care adviser. If videoconferencing is augmented by additional techniques, such as observed examination and digital auscultation, reliable diagnostic data may be obtained remotely.

Commonly, teleconsultation via videoconference is undertaken by the health-care professional responsible for the patient with the aim of seeking decision support for diagnosis and treatment. With increasing scarcity of resources, health-care professionals may not be available in remote areas and video-consultation may involve an appropriately trained lay person or even the patient operating the equipment. An appropriately trained third party will be able to elicit and report examination findings either independently or under the supervision of the base adviser. They may discuss the case with the adviser and administer treatment. Care must be taken during the consultation to include the patient in any discussion. The remote practitioner should be familiar with the data required for the consultation to proceed. The remote user may add his or her own interpretation of the data prior to transfer, which may bias the diagnostic decision of the base adviser. Checklists at both sites may help to minimize error and bias (Figure 9.2).

Direct consultation with the patient allows collection of information with no added interpretation and the visualization of non-verbal prompts. However, this may lengthen the consultation time and will be limited by the patient's ability to describe symptoms or undertake self-examination under the direction of the base adviser. Ideally, a videoconsultation will involve direct interactions with both the patient and the third party. The advising health-care professional must be aware of the importance of involving all participants at the remote site.[14]

Undertaking a videoconsultation

How is a videoconsultation undertaken? First of all, it should be structured: structure facilitates any type of consultation and various systems are taught in communications training. When introducing videoconsultation to a service, most practitioners do not review or alter the structure of their consultation technique (which may contain several bad habits). Reviewing technique and making appropriate changes will greatly enhance the experience of videoconferencing for all participants.

✈ medical advice call form   ⼁ theFirstCall

Serial number for office use only							

Patient Details to be completed by Cabin Crew/Medical Professional

1	Age	2	Gender	A	Male	B	Female

3	Description of Illness/Complaint

4	Conscious Level	A	Alert	B	Verbal	C	Pain	D	Unresponsive
5	Breathing	A	Normal	B	Irregular	C	Noisy	D	Difficult
6	Skin Appearance	A	Normal	B	Pale	C	Flushed	D	Cyanosed
7	Pain	A	None	B	Mild	C	Moderate	D	Severe
8	Pulse Rate								
9	Temperature °C								
10	Allergies		Negative		Affirm	Specify			
11	Taking Medications		Negative		Affirm	Specify			
12	Past Medical History		Negative		Affirm	Specify			
13	Medically Qualified Person Volunteered		Negative		Affirm	Specify			

14	Initial Care Given

Flight Details to be completed by Flight Deck

Additional Details to be completed by Cabin Crew/Medical Professional

15	Aircraft Contact Telephone No.			Patient's Surname		
16	Aircraft Callsign			Patient's Forenames		
17	HF Selcal Callsign			Address		
18	Destination					
19	ETA	GMT			Country	
Divert	Negative	Affirm	Date of Birth		
Ground Based Medical Advice			Today's Date \ \	Hour	Min
			Cabin Crew/Medical Professional		
			Address		
			Relevant Professional Qualification		
			Signature		

Figure 9.2 An example of a checklist: the medical advice form for ground-to-air advice

A structured videoconsultation should involve consideration of:

- environment
- session initiation
- dialogue
- session closure.

Environment

The environment is very important for good-quality consultation. In traditional practice, consulting rooms and equipment are laid out to facilitate good communication with the patient present. Simply adding a videoconferencing unit to this environment is likely to be sub-optimal.

Three factors of the environment should be considered:

(1) planning
(2) equipment
(3) training.

Planning

The location of the videoconferencing equipment is very important. In a facility where advice is given but not sought, the room may be relatively small as only a single health-care professional is likely to be present. Ideally, the room should be in a quiet area. Background noise, which may be so familiar as to go unnoticed by the adviser, will become obvious during videoconferencing.[15]

The ambient lighting in the room must be sufficient to visualize the participants. The colour scheme of the walls visible to the remote site should enhance clarity. Light blue, non-reflective colours have been shown to be suitable. The area visualized during the videoconsultation should not include windows, in order to minimize excess light on sunny days. Access should be controlled in order to minimize interruptions. The advice-giver's site should include a desk, either as an integral part of the videoconferencing set-up or separately to record data on paper or computer (Figure 9.3).

Ideally, the remote videoconferencing unit should be placed in a dedicated, easily accessible, private room with all standard consultation equipment available. This is rarely possible in practice and units are placed in existing multipurpose rooms. For example, remote minor injuries teleconsultations are usually undertaken from small community hospitals or minor injury units.

Additional equipment such as document cameras and digital stethoscopes will need to be accommodated. The room should be long enough to allow examination of the whole patient within a single view of the videocamera. Sockets for telephone lines and electricity should be installed in suitable positions to enable the room to be used to best advantage.

The purpose of the consultation will dictate the setting. For example, in telepsychiatry, the videoconferencing unit need be set up to view only a seated patient but privacy will be paramount. As most remote sites will be consulting on

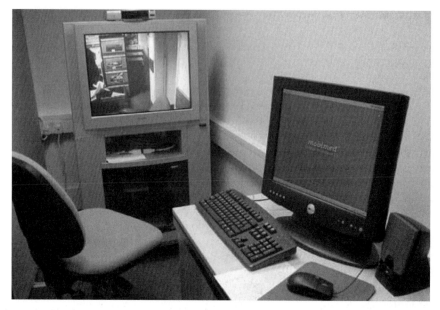

Figure 9.3 A videoconferencing room, illustrating the position of camera and desk

a variety of conditions to different specialist advisers, it is important to build in flexibility. Videoconferencing units may be installed in each consulting area but this is expensive. A better solution may be to install extension points in consulting areas and use a single videoconferencing unit on a moveable trolley. However, the operator will have to be proficient at moving and setting up the equipment.

Creating a designated room for videoconferencing ensures privacy and allows the environment to be optimized. However, it may discourage widespread use of teleconsultation if it is the sole site for videoconferencing. Videoconferencing units should be as widespread as practicable in a variety of settings to encourage usage.

In principle, any health-care professional who is competent clinically and confident in operating telemedicine equipment may be involved in tele-consultations. The majority of teleconsultation applications were initially evaluated on doctor-to-doctor consultations, but it has become clear that the remote health-care provider may come from a variety of backgrounds. For example, teleneurology examinations at remote sites may routinely be undertaken by appropriately trained nursing assistants.[16] Similarly, emergency nurse practitioners (ENPs) may give the majority of advice in minor injuries telemedicine (Figure 9.4).

Equipment

Videoconferencing equipment should be selected for quality of image and ease of use. Simple, intuitive controls are ideal. The majority of teleconsultations require

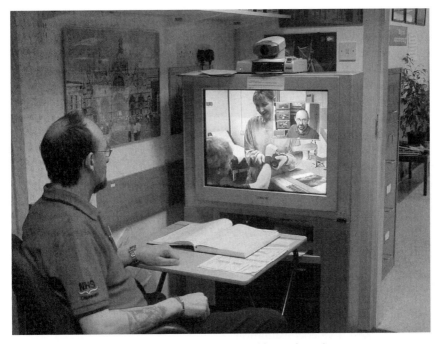

Figure 9.4 Plaster being applied under supervision via videoconferencing

only a few functions. Unfortunately, each new generation of videoconferencing equipment appears to be more and more complex, which tends to discourage practitioners who are not fully conversant with operating it. One solution is to preset the majority of functions and leave visible only those controls necessary to perform a simple teleconsultation.

The equipment should be compatible with the remote site. As international standards have developed, most commercial equipment will interconnect irrespective of the manufacturer. Some remote sites will have older equipment and it is always worth performing test calls before connecting for clinical purposes. The ability to remotely control the remote site's camera is important, especially if the far site has a low volume of use. This allows the base practitioner to adjust the camera view to suit his or her own requirements and assist inexperienced remote users. Storing preset views on the remote site unit may facilitate supervised examination.

Technical support should be easily accessible, especially during normal working hours. This support should include line/network assistance, as well as troubleshooting for videoconferencing equipment. The equipment and its settings should be checked regularly.[14]

Training

Operation of videoconferencing equipment may readily be learned by all grades of staff.[17] However, it is common for practitioners to commence teleconsultations without undertaking training in either the technical or the clinical aspects of the procedure. Technical training should focus on the core functions of the equipment, such as establishing a call, adjusting the camera view and sound volume. Simple aide memoires should be available at all videoconferencing stations to guide the user. Ideally, troubleshooting guides should be in the form of an algorithm.

Clinical training should include which consultations are suitable for video-conference and highlight areas where special considerations may be required. For example, minor linear fractures may be missed on X-ray transmission during minor injury teleconsulting and training should emphasize treatment based on clinical symptoms and signs, even in the presence of a normal X-ray. Training should include mock teleconsultations using clinical scenarios which illustrate videoconferencing technique and potential pitfalls.

Session initiation

Agreed procedures for initiating a teleconsultation should be in place. For non-urgent cases, a booking system should be instigated using appropriate media, such as the telephone or email. For unscheduled conditions, notification of a call may not be required if the volume of calls is sufficient for a base practitioner to be available at all times. However, it is more common for a telephone call to be placed to request a videoconsultation.

Once the call is established, a rapid check should be made to ensure that sound and picture quality is satisfactory at the remote end. Unless it has already been done by the remote practitioner, the purpose and structure of the consultation should be explained to the patient and roles established. Introductions should be made of all participants involved in the consultation. A common error is for the patient to be increasingly ignored as discussion ensues between the two health-care professionals. Patients should be informed that they may contribute at any time.

Dialogue

The teleconsultation should then proceed. Aide memoires at both ends are useful to facilitate this process. A checklist for minor injuries management may also act as a record of the consultation. Care should be taken by all parties to avoid talking over each other. Diction should be clear and emphasized.

The picture-in-picture function should always be used to confirm the image being transmitted to the remote site (Figure 9.5). The camera is of course not in the screen but has to be positioned at some point around the screen, usually above. If the image on the screen is addressed directly, the view sent to the remote site will therefore be off centre. For example, if the camera is mounted above the screen, the operator's gaze should be directed towards the upper part of the screen so that he or she appears to be talking into the camera.

The content and length of the dialogue will be determined by the nature of the medical problem being consulted on. Observation of directed activities such as examination, suturing, plaster application, ultrasound scanning and, in some

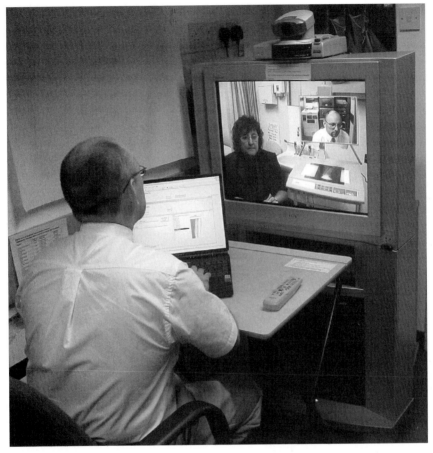

Figure 9.5 Teleconsultation in progress, showing the picture-in-picture function

cases, resuscitative measures may be undertaken. Transmission of additional data such as X-ray films or close-up images using secondary cameras may be required.

Session closure

Once the dialogue stage is complete, the patient and remote health-care practitioner should be asked if they have any questions. Once these are answered, the outcome and any further actions required arising from the consultation are summarized and agreed. Patients should be asked directly if they are satisfied with the consultation. Remote practitioners should be invited to make contact by telephone if they have any unanswered queries. This allows matters to be discussed which may not have been suitable to air in the presence of the patient, such as sensitive diagnoses or practical problems with the equipment. At this point, the connection should be terminated and any remaining contemporaneous notes completed.[18]

Troubleshooting

Occasionally, unexpected problems will arise during the most well prepared teleconsultations. Minor problems with picture quality or sound, which were not sufficiently severe to stop the consultation, must be corrected on completion or reported to technical support staff. Commonly, such problems go unaddressed, causing difficulties with subsequent sessions.

Table 9.1 Troubleshooting guide

Problem	Solution
No sound	Turn up the television volume
Remote site unable to hear	Check the mute button
No picture	Check the input selection
Call cutting out	Reboot the system

A troubleshooting guide of common problems and their solutions should be readily available at each site (see Table 9.1). A contingency plan for total failure of the system should be in place. This may include using a secondary videoconferencing site, rescheduling the consultation or transferring the patient to the main facility. Frequently, individuals who are reluctant to undertake teleconsultation cite fear of medicolegal issues, but there is little evidence of significant problems arising directly from the use of teleconsultation (see Chapter 11).

Conclusion

An increase in the use of teleconsultation is expected in the future, due to clinical need. Increasingly robust and affordable technology will facilitate this. Selection of the appropriate medium for the purpose of the consultation should be undertaken. Recognizing the advantages and limitations of the available media, combined with appropriate planning and training, will maximize the utilization of teleconsultations.

References

1   Howie JG, Heaney D, Maxwell M. Quality, core values and the general practice consultation: issues of definition, measurement and delivery. *Fam Pract* 2004;**21**:458–68
2   Benschoter RA, Wittson CL, Ingham CG. Teaching and consultation by television. I. Closed-circuit collaboration. *Ment Hosp* 1995;**16**:99–100
3   Benger JR, Noble SM, Coast J, Kendall JM. The safety and effectiveness of minor injuries telemedicine. *Emerg Med J* 2004;**21**:438–45
4   *Securing Future Practice. Shaping the new Medical Workforce for Scotland.* Edinburgh: Scottish Executive, 2004. See http://www.scotland.gov.uk/library5/health/sfpnmw.pdf (last checked 30 March 2005)

5   Pedley DK, Bissett K, Connolly EM, *et al.* Prospective observational cohort study of time saved by prehospital thrombolysis for ST elevation myocardial infarction delivered by paramedics. *BMJ* 2003;**327**:22–6

6   Thorson H, Witt K, Hollnagel H, Multerad K. The purpose of the general practice consultation from the patient's perspective: theoretical aspects. *Fam Pract* 2001;**18**:638–43

7   Eedy DJ, Wootton R. Teledermatology: a review. *Br J Dermatol* 2001;**144**:696–707

8   Harno KS. Telemedicine in managing demand for secondary-care services. *J Telemed Telecare* 1999;**5**:189–92

9   Patterson V, Humphreys J, Chua R. Email triage of new neurological outpatient referrals from general practice. *J Neurol Neurosurg Psychiatry* 2004;**75**:617–20

10 Schwaab B, Katalinic A, Ridel J, Sheikhzadeh A. Prehospital diagnosis of myocardial ischaemia by telecardiology: safety and efficiency of a 12 lead electrocardiogram recorded and transmitted by the patient. *J Telemed Telecare* 2005;**11**:41–4

11 Ward S. NHS Direct: Dial M for …. medical advice. *Health Serv J* 2001;**111**:24–6

12 Braun RP, Vecchietti JL, Thomas L, *et al.* Telemedical wound care using a new generation of mobile telephones: a feasibility study. *Arch Dermatol* 2005;**141**:254–8

13 Aujla K, Nag R, Ferguson J, Howell M, Cahill C. Rationalizing radio medical advice for maritime emergencies. *J Telemed Telecare* 2003;**9** (Suppl. 1):12–14

14 Miller EA. The technical and interpersonal aspects of telemedicine: effects on doctor–patient communication. *J Telemed Telecare* 2003;**9**:1–7

15 Major J. Telemedicine room design. *J Telemed Telecare* 2005;**11**:10–14

16 Chua R, Craig J, Wootton R, Patterson V. Randomised controlled trial of telemedicine for new neurological outpatient referrals. *J Neurol Neurosurg Psychiatry* 2001;**71**:63–6

17 Padgham K, Scott J, Krichell A, McEachen T, Hislop L. Misconceptions surrounding videoconferencing. *J Telemed Telecare* 2005;**11** (Suppl. 1):61–2

18 Lian P, Chong R, Zhai X, Ning Y. The quality of medical records in teleconsultation. *J Telemed Telecare* 2003;**9**:35–41

Further information

1   Baruffaldi F, Gualdrini G, Toni A. Comparison of asynchronous and realtime teleconsulting for orthopaedic second opinions. *J Telemed Telecare* 2002;**8**:297–301

2   Jaatinen PT, Forsstrom J, Loula P. Teleconsultations: who uses them and how? *J Telemed Telecare* 2002;**8**:319–24

3   Tachakra S, Newson R, Wootton R, Stinson A. Avoiding artificiality in teleconsultations. *J Telemed Telecare* 2001;**7** (Suppl. 1):39–42

Section 4: Other Aspects of Telemedicine

►10

Benefits and drawbacks of telemedicine

N M Hjelm

Introduction

Telemedicine is a vast subject, but as yet there are limited data on the clinical effectiveness and cost-effectiveness of most telemedicine applications. As a result, objective information about the benefits and drawbacks of telemedicine is limited. This review is therefore based mainly on preliminary results, opinions and predictions.

Many potential benefits of telemedicine can be envisaged, including:

- improved access to information;
- provision of care not previously deliverable;
- improved access to services and increasing care delivery;
- improved professional education;
- quality control of screening programmes;
- reduced health-care costs.

Improved access to information

Telemedicine can improve access to information for health professionals, for patients and for the population in general.

Information for health professionals
Electronic search engines such as MEDLARS, PUBMED and others have laid the foundation for a silent revolution that enables any health professional to have access to up-to-date 'case-oriented' information within seconds, via the Internet. Wireless computer connections mean that searches can even be conducted at the bedside. Full copies of articles in journals and books can be ordered and received as an attachment to an email message from a distant reference library. This application of telemedicine provides the basis for daily, continuous education, which should expand and maintain the skills of health professionals at all levels. The benefits of this application of telemedicine are obvious and cannot be overestimated.

Communication between health professionals
Communication between the primary and secondary health-care sectors has traditionally been carried out by mail, but email is increasingly being used for this

purpose. As a result, information kept in a computerized data file can be attached to an email message, permitting easy and instantaneous transfer of patient information between general practitioners (GPs) and hospitals. Health professionals in primary care can access patient records, kept in databases of individual hospitals, groups of hospitals or entire health regions, ensuring, for example, that hospital discharge letters are made available without delay.

Information for patients and the general population

In many countries, computers in schools, homes, work-places and local libraries allow electronically stored information to be accessed through the Internet. This has provided an opportunity to establish a 'super-highway' to information about health and disease, which can be used for many purposes:

- *To provide information to patients* – for understanding the nature of their disease, its prognosis, the reasons for carrying out certain investigations and the effect that any treatment might have. Once patients have acquired such knowledge, it could provide the basis for shared decision-making between patients and health professionals,[1] empowering patients and encouraging self-help. It is therefore crucial that information is accurate and case-oriented (though see below under 'Drawbacks').
- *To provide information to the general public* – in particular to the disadvantaged/under-served, for example as part of health promotion or health education to people, schools and health-care centres. This could turn out to be the most cost-effective way of improving knowledge about health and disease, and the relationship between lifestyle and the quality of life. In practice, however, the value of this method of providing information will ultimately depend on the quality and presentation of the information (see below under 'Drawbacks').

Multimedia presentations on health and disease can also be considered to be telemedicine. Such presentations have the potential to overcome problems with illiteracy. However, they are often futuristic in their approach and may raise unrealistic expectations among the general population. Sensible and directed presentations, supplemented with additional information, for example, via the Internet, may redress some of the past and present difficulties associated with some of these presentations.

Provision of care not previously deliverable

In the 1980s, the Norwegian government initiated a national telemedicine programme. The main reason was to offer citizens in small, rural communities an alternative to travel, because of local deficiencies in specialist care. Overall, this political initiative has been vindicated[2] and has been replicated subsequently in other parts of the world, including Australia, Canada, Greece, Japan and the USA.

Considered from this socioeconomic perspective, telemedicine has contributed to providing health care to previously under-served regions. However, the effect of telemedicine on delivering care in a local context, i.e. within a community or even within a hospital, should also be considered. There is the potential for telemedicine to have an even greater impact in these environments because of the much larger number of medical episodes that would be likely to occur. Such applications of telemedicine have only recently been considered.[3]

Improved access to services and increasing care delivery

For many years, the telephone has been extensively used by health professionals and patients for keeping in touch. This is widely viewed as an effective form of telemedicine. Advances in communications technology have, however, increased the potential methods and speed by which health-care professionals and patients can communicate. Expected benefits of such improvements in communication are:

- faster access to the health professional;
- increased convenience, and time savings for patients;
- improved equity of access to care between and within regions, previously denied because of such factors as socioeconomic constraints, especially in countries in the developing world, and the tendency for specialized services to be centralized in urban centres;
- improved access between and within primary, secondary and tertiary care;
- improved quality of care.

Telemedicine may improve access in primary care and in secondary care.

Improved access in primary care
In primary care, telemedicine may facilitate communication with the GP; it may also improve access for patients at home.

GP consultations
Many consultations in a GP's surgery relate to minor ailments such as respiratory and gastrointestinal infections, back pain and renewal of prescriptions. Once the diagnosis has been established, the effect of treatment needs to be monitored. This could be provided by videolink. Additional prescriptions could be sent via the Internet to a nearby pharmacy, which would arrange for delivery to the patient. Such an approach could be beneficial for patients, especially if they were not well enough to travel. It could also be beneficial for the health professional, as the teleconsultation could take place at any time, and for the pharmacy, as its dispensing service could be better planned. There is evidence that such an approach could work.[4]

Home monitoring and treatment

Home monitoring and treatment of patients suffering from a wide range of diseases would improve the quality of care and be more efficient. The five examples given below illustrate how telemedicine could facilitate such improvements.

(1) *Diabetes*

Patients with diabetes mellitus need regular monitoring in order to minimize long-term complications. Diabetes mellitus is increasingly being diagnosed in younger patients with busy work schedules and other commitments. Traditionally, monitoring has required regular visits to outpatient clinics, which are often time-consuming and can result in substantial interference to a busy work or home schedule. Much could be gained by providing at least part of the monitoring required by such means as teleconsultation. This would minimize the effect of medical intervention on daily life, and provide an opportunity for health professionals to observe patients in their homes, potentially more frequently than at present.

To augment the above, assays are now available to allow home testing of blood and urine glucose levels (Figure 10.1). If performed correctly, the results of such assays can be as accurate as those carried out in specialist laboratories, although in practice the results of tests carried out by patients often differ from those performed in laboratories.[5] This is not surprising as patients usually lack the training required to carry out laboratory investigations. However, this situation could be substantially improved if health professionals used the teleconsulting equipment to observe how patients carry out the tests. Glucose analysers could also be linked to the telephone, transmitting the results of tests performed to the health professional's office. This option could potentially be used both for monitoring the frequency and outcome of tests carried out by the patient, and for registering the results obtained from control samples sent to the patient's home to check the accuracy of the analyser.

(2) *Hypertension*

One important reason why patients suffering from high blood pressure visit health professionals is to have their blood pressure taken. As electronic blood pressure monitors are now available, patients can measure their own blood pressure and transmit the results, for example, to their GP, by telephone. Prescriptions of medication could subsequently be based on the transmitted results and arranged as discussed above. It might be expected that such an approach, where blood pressure measurements are taken at home and work, would result in the recording of more representative blood pressure readings, and might even reduce the number of patients with 'white-coat' hypertension. To ensure that readings were being accurately recorded, patients could initially be supervised using an inexpensive audiovisual link.[6]

(3) *Home deliveries*

In industrialized countries, there has been an increase in the number of home deliveries over the last decade. Although only uncomplicated pregnancies are recommended for home delivery, complications can still occur. In such situations,

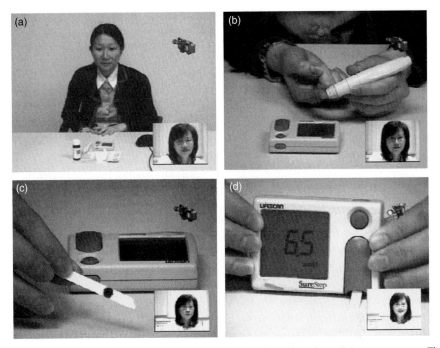

Figure 10.1 Monitoring blood glucose measurements as part of a telemedicine programme. The patient (a) is taking capillary blood (b), showing the test strip with blood (c), and the final result (d). The supervising laboratory technician appears in the lower right-hand corner of the monitor (Photo credit: NM Hjelm)

midwives could potentially receive immediate advice from an obstetrician in a secondary care institution using an interactive videolink. Such measures, although clearly not a substitute for high-quality specialized care, might improve the quality of service in some scenarios, to the benefit of both mother and neonate, as well as providing the midwife with continuous professional education. It is likely that developing countries would benefit even more from having access to monitoring of home deliveries, partly because the incidence of complications in these countries is higher.[7]

(4) *Home nursing, care for the elderly and chronically ill*

It is important that the mental and physical needs of the elderly and chronically ill are supported, so that they can continue to remain out of hospitals and other institutions for as long as possible, despite having age-related handicaps and illnesses. This can improve their quality of life, as well as reduce the costs of prolonged stays in community and hospital care facilities (Figure 10.2). The installation of home monitoring systems that could monitor physiological variables, such as the electrocardiogram (ECG) and blood pressure, and videolinks that would allow health professionals and relatives to interact more

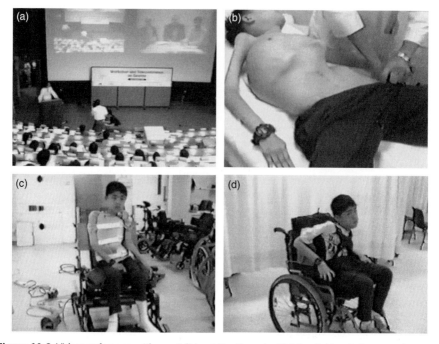

Figure 10.2 Videoconference with specialists at the Toronto Children's Hospital concerning a wheelchair for a severely handicapped child in Hong Kong. (a) The conference room with the Toronto specialists to the right on the screen; (b) the patient (deformed chest due to Duchenne's disease, requiring support in the wheelchair for breathing; (c) early stage in building the wheelchair; (d) the patient on his way into the conference room (Photo credit: NM Hjelm)

frequently with the elderly, could go some way to achieving this. In effect, a 'virtual home' for the elderly and their relatives could be developed, which would permit relatives to take more responsibility for caring without having to compromise their own commitments. Such measures could also help to diminish the reportedly high incidence of abuse of the elderly[8] by creating a more open, safer and happier virtual environment for institutionalized care.

(5) *Dialysis*

In the past, patients with renal failure have had regular dialysis treatment in hospitals on a day-patient basis. This has been very time-consuming for patients, for example preventing them from continuing their employment or applying for daytime jobs. Home dialysis under the supervision of a dialysis centre using a videolink could provide a solution to this problem for many patients, improving their quality of life and allowing them to work regular hours.[9] It is also likely that dialysis centres could monitor more patients by such techniques. The obvious advantage of a videolink is that staff at the dialysis centre can observe how patients are handling the dialysis equipment and guide the patients in case of complications.

Improved access in secondary care

Telemedicine may improve access to hospitals. It may also improve access both between and within hospitals.

Emergency specialist support

An example of an emergency situation that might benefit from use of a videolink is a major traffic accident involving a number of cars on a busy road, all lanes being blocked in both directions by damaged and queuing cars, preventing access by ambulances. In such a situation, health professionals could still reach the site of the accident by motorcycle or helicopter. A portable audiovisual system, transmitting perhaps by microwave,[10] would permit links with the nearest accident and emergency (A&E) department. Although there are still technical problems to solve, the same type of equipment installed in an ambulance could also provide a similar service both to victims of accidents and other emergency situations, and improve the quality of care during the transport of the victim(s). As ambulances are often staffed with health professionals trained in emergency medicine they could, under the supervision of specialists in the A&E department, be more interventionist in their approach during transit.

Similar services by videolink have already been established for emergency situations at sea, on aircraft and as part of rescue operations in major civil disasters.[11] The US Navy has many vessels equipped with videolinks, enabling the general surgeons on board to link up with specialist centres by satellite for advice about how to handle complicated injuries.[12] In the case of a major civil disaster, similar services could be provided by a mobile audiovisual system, carried to the site of the disaster by a helicopter. The helicopter could also function as a relay station for the telecommunications required.

Shared care for diagnosis and treatment

Shared care is important in providing optimum care and best use of resources. Full-scale implementation of shared care would be facilitated using videolinks, allowing patients, primary health professionals and health specialists to meet in a virtual clinic.[13] The potential of this approach is that a teleconsultation can be carried out from the GP's surgery to the specialist centre. This would result in fewer delays between decisions being taken at the specialist centre and action occurring, save time for patients and health professionals, and provide ongoing educational opportunities for those in primary care. However, it has to be said that the costs and benefits of such schemes remain to be established.

Inter-hospital access

Many medium-sized hospitals provide 24 h cover for specialist services while others provide only a skeleton service. Telemedicine could substantially improve this situation and reduce disparities in the level of cover between institutions. In radiology, there are already many hospitals where images are taken locally by a radiographer and then transmitted electronically to a radiologist somewhere else, for interpretation. Since there is a much larger pool of specialists at the specialist

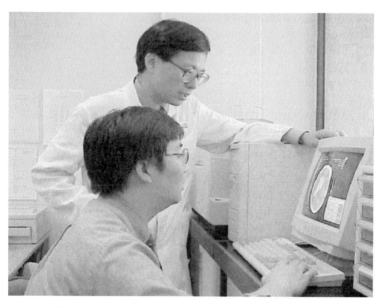

Figure 10.3 Teleradiology. Transmission of computerized tomography scans to a neurosurgery centre allows an informed decision to be made about the merits of transfer. The transmitting and receiving centres can view the same image on their monitors and use the telephone for comments (Photo credit: NM Hjelm)

hospital than the smaller hospitals can muster, the quality of service is undoubtedly improved (Figure 10.3). The obvious advantages to the local radiologists are more regular working hours and continuous education. It is estimated that this new system is no more expensive than the old one.

The provision of specialist services to manage inpatients, at district general and other small hospitals that do not have specialists on site, by teleconsultation has also been tried. In many specialties, it has been shown to be an effective way of providing high-quality care that otherwise would not be available, e.g. in psychiatry.[14]

Intra-hospital access

So far, apart from applications for teaching purposes, there are few reported examples of telemedicine applications that improve intra-hospital access. However, there is a precedent for this in the telephone, which is already extensively used to provide many services, ranging from interpretation of laboratory investigations to a second opinion about a patient. There is no doubt that the effectiveness of these consultations is often restricted by the absence of the visual element, limiting the ability of health professionals to make accurate clinical decisions without seeing, for example, the radiological image or the patient. As a result, busy health professionals lose much time rushing up and down the stairs of large hospital complexes or queuing in front of elevators, in an

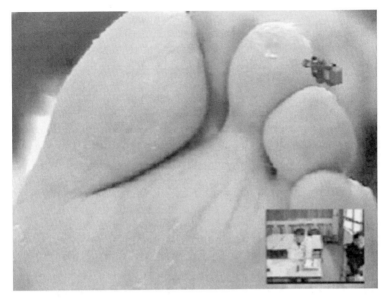

Figure 10.4 Telemedicine assessment of a woman in Hong Kong with gout, complaining about pain in her left foot. The examining physician in a geriatric hospital is seen in the lower right corner of the photograph. No specific therapy was required except asking the patient to put on warmer socks (Photo credit: NM Hjelm)

attempt to reach patients quickly. The introduction of an audiovisual infrastructure in the hospital setting that could link wards, operating theatres, clinical service departments and doctors' offices by a local broadband network might considerably improve this situation. For example, by using videolinks:

- surgeons and pathologists could discuss the best site from which to take a tissue biopsy and jointly review any frozen section taken;
- consultants could supervise junior medical staff, providing them with a second opinion on wards, in outpatient clinics and the A&E department;[15]
- pathologists and radiologists could provide an immediate service 'at the point of care'.[16,17]

In general, it can be predicted that in hospitals the audiovisual presentation of information will gradually replace the telephone as a more cost-effective means of bridging 'short distances' (Figure 10.4).

Improved professional education

The provision of undergraduate, postgraduate and continuing training by electronic means has proved to be highly successful.[18,19] Many undergraduate students use a laptop computer from the day they begin their first course, for such activities as downloading printed materials, videos and tutorials, and accessing medical information.

At the postgraduate level, examples abound of telemedical applications being used for the purpose of education. Examples include the self-test applications for some specialties that can be accessed on the Internet, the ability to access lectures given by distant specialists using videoconferencing facilities, and more recently the setting of simulators for teaching practical skills, such as intubation for anaesthetists and endoscopy for surgeons. Examination of undergraduate and postgraduate students by videolink has also been conducted, saving the school travel expenses and the examiner travelling time.

It is safe to predict that telemedical education will rapidly become an integral part of the teaching curriculum for most health professionals, improving their access to a wide range of courses of the highest quality. For example, three-dimensional images of a joint or a skull could be downloaded, allowing surgeons to acquire manipulative skills by practising on the virtual image using real surgical tools. Downloading a virtual patient could provide health professionals with an opportunity to develop their consultative skills.[20]

Quality control of screening programmes

The success of mass screening programmes, such as those used for the detection of breast cancer and cervical cancer, depends on the use of specific and sensitive methods, which give reproducible results in all centres carrying out the tests, over long periods of time. Usually, external quality control programmes achieve this via the postal distribution of radiological images and pathological slides, for example. Using the Internet and other more advanced telecommunications methods for distribution has been shown to result in a much faster turnaround than is possible in conventional quality control programmes. Such programmes could, however, also be enhanced by using other modern methods of communication, which might include realtime demonstrations of images transmitted by videolink to participating sites from a dedicated centre.[17]

In the UK, recent events have indicated that a national register is required to monitor the outcome of advanced surgery, e.g. cardiac surgery. An additional measure, however, could be that external specialists provide realtime advice by videolink during the operative procedures. Such an approach has been tried successfully for endoscopic surgery.[18]

Reduced health-care costs

Large-scale trials have yet to be carried out for most telemedical applications. As a result, there is little quantitative information about the savings resulting from using telemedicine instead of traditional methods of providing care. So far most applications have focused on bridging large distances, caring for patients in remote or inaccessible areas. Such applications are often quite expensive because of the prevailing telecommunications costs.

In the long term, telemedicine could dramatically reduce the overall costs of health services because of its potential to allow a fundamental restructuring of the way health care is delivered. This would principally result from redistributing resources from the hospital environment into primary care. Providing more services in primary care and ultimately in patients' homes could be considered to be the ultimate goal for health-care delivery and in part this could be facilitated by telemedicine.

Drawbacks

Although telemedicine clearly has a wide range of potential benefits, it also has some disadvantages. The main drawbacks of telemedicine that can be envisaged are:

- a breakdown in the relationship between health professional and patient;
- a breakdown in the relationship between health professionals;
- issues concerning the quality of health information;
- organizational and bureaucratic difficulties.

Breakdown in the relationship between health professional and patient

It should not be assumed *a priori* that the use of teleconsultations will result in a breakdown in the patient–doctor relationship. The telephone has functioned very well as a communications medium without any documented indications of it decreasing the quality of the communication between patient and doctor. Teleconsultation may even improve the relationship, for example in matters concerning sexuality and family problems, where a psychological 'safety distance' may make the patient more open and forthcoming.[21] Therefore, the risk of breakdown in the relationship from using a videolink might relate more to communicative skills and lack of formal training in using telemedical equipment rather than the format of the communication itself (see below under 'Depersonalization'). However, more research is required if the optimum procedure for interacting with patients by videolink is to be established.

Factors which might cause a breakdown in the relationship between health professional and patient compared with normal face-to-face consultations are:

- physical and mental factors;
- depersonalization;
- different process of consultation;
- inability to perform the whole consultation;
- reduced confidence of patients and health professionals;
- different knowledge and skills required of health professionals and ergonomic issues.

Physical and mental factors

Patients suffering from reduced vision or who are hard of hearing are likely to have some difficulty following the information presented in a video consultation. It seems, however, that by displaying questions as text and using sign language, these limitations can be overcome.[22] Videoconsultations have been successfully carried out with disabled patients.[23]

Depersonalization

During a teleconsultation, the images of both the health-care worker and the patient are projected onto a monitor and all interactions between the two parties are indirect. As our perceptions of what is seen on a monitor are very much influenced by our experience of watching TV, a teleconsultation might not be experienced as being real by either party. There is anecdotal evidence that elderly patients at times do not accept that a physician, appearing on what looks like a TV screen, can see and listen to them properly. In one instance, a resident in an old people's home participating in a trial asked the female research assistant sitting next to her to repeat what was said by the male physician on the monitor, and finally asked the research assistant, 'Why are you talking to me in a man's voice?' (Hjelm *et al.*, unpublished work).

Different process of consultation

During face-to-face and telephone consultations, patients and health professionals introduce themselves in a natural way as part of the consultation, and in doing so secure the identity of both parties. However, it is observed that this important introductory step is often omitted during a videoconsultation. The reason for this omission is uncertain but could perhaps be explained by technical distractions or it may reflect the fact that when watching TV, the identity of the actors is often not important for understanding what is going on.

Both health professionals and patients should be asked to identify themselves at the start of a telemedicine session and the patient should be told briefly about the technical aspects of the session and asked about the quality of the audiovisual transmission. How to improve 'bedside manners' during a video-consultation is included in Chapter 9.

Inability to perform the whole consultation

A videoconsultation is limited by the fact that the entire physical examination cannot be carried out over a videolink. This particularly applies to examinations where palpation is an important component. In such cases, the specialist has to rely on the findings of another health-care worker, whose examination of the patient they have witnessed and, in practice, this often seems to be satisfactory. These limitations may gradually be removed by future technological developments, which will allow the investigator to carry out examinations indirectly that at present are impossible.

Confidence of patients and health professionals

In general, patients seem satisfied with most telemedicine applications, including teleconsultation,[24] and health professionals have expressed confidence in using, for example, videolinks, for providing care.[25] There is however some scepticism about the use of telemedicine, if not open hostility to it, among a proportion of health professionals. Evidence gained from properly conducted clinical trials is likely to be the only way to change such opinions.

Different knowledge and skills required of health professionals and ergonomic issues

There is no doubt that the equipment required for telemedicine can sometimes be daunting to use. It is therefore essential, if users are not to be scared off, that sensible presentations of the applications are given, that do not overemphasize to the users what are essentially irrelevant technical details. During these presentations, the skills required to operate the equipment should be taught. This is particularly important because at present there are few commercial video systems available at a reasonable price for dedicated use in the medical environment. Health-care professionals should therefore encourage the industrial sector to develop such systems according to their specifications. It is also important that the limitations of the equipment used are detailed. Some universities already offer *ad hoc* courses in telemedicine but such courses need to be incorporated, in the longer term, into the undergraduate curriculum of all health professionals.

Breakdown in the relationship between health professionals

This is an area that has not been explored to any great extent, although there is the risk that highly skilled staff at the remote site will perceive that their autonomy is threatened by the use of telemedicine, or worse still that they will become no more than technicians, acting solely as the hands of the specialist, who will receive all the plaudits for performing a consultation.

Issues concerning the quality of health information

As indicated above and in other chapters, there is a wealth of medical information available via the Internet. This can be broadly divided into three categories:

- textbook-style information, produced by medical schools and other academic institutions;
- abstracts of peer-reviewed articles or whole articles in biomedical journals;
- health pamphlets and articles intended for the general public, produced by individuals, charitable organizations or special-interest groups.

It is the information in the third category that gives the greatest reasons for concern, as far as patients and other non-health-care professionals are concerned, because the content can be biased, inaccurate, confusing and misleading for a patient seeking information about a particular condition. As with all printed information, medical information on the Internet should contain relevant, research-based data in a form that is acceptable and useful to patients. To facilitate this, guidelines should be worked out for the production of medical information directed at patients and the general public; this might involve including a review process and a 'kitemark' to indicate that the information is accurate and meets recognized standards (see Chapter 12 for further information).

Problems with the wealth of information available can, however, also affect the health-care professional. This principally arises not because of quality but because of the seemingly endless quantity of information available. The concept of information overload is already a reality for many health-care professionals, since it appears to be impossible to keep up to date with developments. This is also the case in the telemedicine field, as witnessed by the huge increase in publications on the subject.

Organizational and bureaucratic difficulties

The fact that telemedicine might have great potential for improving health-care delivery does not necessarily mean that it will be implemented. In fact there is little evidence that manufacturers, who are able to develop and manufacture suitable commercial products, politicians, who could promote an environment where funding would be available, health administrators, who could change existing health-care delivery systems, or health professionals, who could guide and implement such changes, are particularly interested in doing so.

The (US) Western Governors' Association Telemedicine Action Report in 1994 listed six 'telemedicine barriers' that could hinder the implementation of this method of health-care delivery:

(1) problems with infrastructure planning and development;
(2) problems with telecommunications regulations;
(3) problems with reimbursement for telemedicine services, because of absent or inconsistent policies;
(4) problems with licensure and credentialing, because of conflicting interests with regard to ensuring quality of care, regulating professional activities and implementing health policies;
(5) problems with medical malpractice liability, because of uncertainties with regard to the legal status of telemedicine within and between states;
(6) problems with confidentiality, because of the increased risk of unauthorized access to patient information compared with information on paper (this and other legal considerations are discussed in Chapter 11).

The report was updated in 1998,[26] but overall, little progress had been made to eliminate barriers 1, 2, 3 and 5. Furthermore, barrier 4 had, if anything, been raised, even though barrier 6 had in effect been eliminated, because electronic transmission of patient information can now be considered to be as safe as conventional methods of information transfer. The lack of progress over a four-year period indicates that much work still remains to be carried out both in the USA and elsewhere in the world before an integrated master plan for telemedicine based on political, professional and economic consensus will emerge.

Other difficulties in implementing telemedicine are likely to arise in trying to convince health-care workers that they should change the way in which they work. The reasons for resistance to change are manifold but include, in addition to those points detailed in the (US) Western Governors' Association Telemedicine Action Report of 1994:

- Lack of evidence as yet for the efficacy or cost-effectiveness of most telemedicine applications. The solution to this is therefore to evaluate any telemedicine application properly.[27–30]
- Perceived threat to the role and status of health-care workers.
- Fear that telemedicine will only increase the current workload of health-care workers, especially in any transitional phase.
- Fear that telemedicine is market-driven, rather than being user-driven, with the risk of market-driven abandonment of products and technologies.
- Fear of technological obsolescence resulting from rapid technological advances.
- Lack of consideration of knowledge and skills of users.
- Cultural and linguistic differences.
- Lack of agreed standards.

Many of the above points are included in the concept of clinical risks related to telemedicine. These are dependent on the level of skills among health professionals and the documented reliability of techniques and procedures used for either diagnostic or interventional purposes. At present, most health professionals are not trained in telemedicine, and there is still little hard evidence for the efficacy or otherwise of telemedicine applications. Therefore, research into obtaining information about the clinical risks associated with telemedicine should be assessed.

Conclusion

Telemedicine has the potential to augment conventional methods of health care so that one day high-quality health care will be available to everyone, everywhere. How telemedicine might achieve this is principally by increasing equitable access to health information and by improving its exchange throughout the entire health-care pyramid. Such a vision will only be possible, however, if telemedicine development is dictated by health needs, if all applications are properly evaluated, and if they are then integrated into the overall health infrastructure.

On balance, the benefits of telemedicine are substantial, assuming that more research will reduce or eliminate the obvious drawbacks.

References

1   Coulter A, Entwistle V, Gilbert D. Sharing decisions with patients: is the information good enough? *BMJ* 1999;**318**:318–22

2   Elford DR. Telemedicine in northern Norway. *J Telemed Telecare* 1997;**3**:1–22

3   Hjelm NM, Lee JC, Cheng D, Chui C. Wiring a medical school and teaching hospital for telemedicine. *Int J Med Inform* 2002;**65**:161–6

4   Gulliford SM, Schneider JK, Jorgenson JA. Using telemedicine technology for pharmaceutical services to ambulatory care patients. *Am J Health-Syst Pharm* 1998;**55**:1512–15

5   Kristensen GB, Nerhus K, Thue G, Sandberg S. Standardized evaluation of instruments for self-monitoring of blood glucose by patients and a technologist. *Clin Chem* 2004;**50**:1068–71

6   Zhang Y, Bai J, Zhou X, *et al.* First trial of home ECG and blood pressure telemonitoring system in Macau. *Telemed J* 1997;**3**:67–72

7   Dyke T, Keake G. The St John Ambulance Service in Port Moresby: a ten-year review, 1984–1993. *Papua New Guinea Med J* 1996;**39**:105–10

8   Tonks A, Bennett G. Elder abuse. *BMJ* 1999;**318**:278

9   Mitchell JG, Disney AP. Clinical applications of renal telemedicine. *J Telemed Telecare* 1997;**3**:158–162

10 Pavlopoulos S, Kyriacou E, Berler A, Dembeyiotis S, Koutsouris D. A novel emergency telemedicine system based on wireless communication technology – AMBULANCE. *IEEE Trans Inform Technol Biomed* 1999;**2**:261–7

11 Rizzo N, Fulvio S, Camerucci S, Carvalho M, Biagini M, Dauri A. Telemedicine for airline passengers, seafarers and islanders. *J Telemed Telecare* 1997;**3** (Suppl. 1):7–9

12 Chimiak WJ, Rainer RO, Chimiak JM, Martinez R. An architecture for naval medicine. *IEEE Trans Inform Technol Biomed* 1997;**1**:73–9

13 Branger P, van't Hooft A, van der Wouden HC. Coordinating shared care using electronic data interchange. *Medinfo* 1995;**8**:1669

14 Hawker F, Kavanagh S, Yellowlees P, Kalucy RS. Telepsychiatry in South Australia. *J Telemed Telecare* 1998;**4**:187–94

15 Tachakra S, Sivakumar A, Everard R, Mullett S, Freij R. Remote trauma management – setting up a system. *J Telemed Telecare* 1996;**2** (Suppl. 1):65–8

16 Eide TJ, Nordrum I. Frozen section service via the telenetwork in northern Norway. *Zentralblatt Pathol* 1992;**138**:409–12

17 Leong FJW-M, Graham AK, McGee JO'D, Schwarzmann P. Clinical trials of robotic interactive telepathology accuracy in the UK breast pathology external quality assurance scheme. *J Telemed Telecare* 1999;**5** (Suppl. 1):139–40

18 Chung SC, Li SS, Poon KO. Teleconferencing in endoscopic surgery. *Hong Kong Med J* 1998;**4**:296–9

19 Jameson DG, O'Hanlon P, Buckton S, Hobsley M. Broadband telemedicine: teaching on the information superhighway. *J Telemed Telecare* 1995;**1**:111–16

20 Richards B, Colman AW, Hollingsworth RA. The current and future role of the Internet in patient education. *Int J Med Inform* 1998;**50**: 279–85

21 Frank AP, Wandell MG, Headings MD, Conant MA, Woody GE, Michel C. Anonymous HIV testing using home collection and telemedicine counseling. A multicenter evaluation. *Arch Intern Med* 1997;**157**:309–14

22 Steinberg AG, Lipton DS, Eckhardt EA, Goldstein M, Sullivan VJ. The diagnostic interview schedule for deaf patients on interactive video: a preliminary investigation. *Am J Psychiatry* 1998;**155**: 1603–4

23 Alimandi L, Andrich R, Porqueddu B. Teleworking in connection with technical aids for disabled persons. *J Telemed Telecare* 1995;**1**:165–72

24 Loane MA, Bloomer SE, Corbett R, *et al.* Patient satisfaction with realtime teledermatology in Northern Ireland. *J Telemed Telecare* 1998;**4**:36–40

25 Sheng OR, Hu PJ, Chau PY, *et al.* A survey of physicians' acceptance of telemedicine. *J Telemed Telecare* 1998;**4** (Suppl. 1):100–2

26 Western Governors Association Telemedicine Reports 1998. See http://www.westgov.org/wga/publicat/combar4.htm (last checked 31 October 2004)

27 Hjelm NM. *Will Telemedicine Run? Hospital Management International Yearbook.* London: International Hospital Federation, SPG Media, 2004:32–3

28 Grigsby B. *2004 TRC Report on US Telemedicine Activity.* Kingston, NJ: Civic Research Institute, 2004

29 Hersh WR, Helfand M, Wallace J, *et al.* Clinical outcomes resulting from telemedicine interventions: a systematic review. *BMC Med Inform Decision Making* 2001;**1**:5

30 Hailey D, Crowe B. A profile of success and failure in telehealth – evidence and opinion from the Success and Failures in Telehealth conferences. *J Telemed Telecare* 2003;**9** (Suppl. 2):22–4

▶11

Legal and ethical aspects of telemedicine

Benedict Stanberry

Introduction

Research into the legal and ethical aspects of telemedicine has been taking place since the mid-1990s. In the UK, one of the first attempts to describe the legal framework for telemedicine was that of Brahams, who stated that 'unforeseen medico-legal implications of telemedicine will be revealed by litigation as it arises'.[1] Brahams identified three core issues of concern: the responsibilities and potential liabilities of the health professional, the duty to maintain the confidentiality and privacy of patient records, and the jurisdictional problems associated with cross-border consultations. Meanwhile, in the US these three issues were also receiving attention, with much concern being reserved for jurisdictional issues because the licensing of doctors in the US takes place on a state-by-state basis, preventing health professionals in one state from providing care in another state via a telemedicine service.

A fourth subject of concern – the reimbursement of care provided using a telemedicine service – was also raised as a problem in the US.[2] European and North American health-care systems differ widely and hence the effects of reimbursement and funding policies on telemedicine services differ from country to country. Regardless of the way in which health care is paid for, however, ensuring that health-care providers are paid for their services when those services are delivered remotely, rather than in the conventional face-to-face manner, is a key issue that must be addressed before telemedicine services can achieve widespread implementation.

In this chapter the generic legal and ethical issues associated with the delivery of telemedicine services are reviewed under 10 separate headings, as summarized in Table 11.1.

Ethical fundamentals

There are a number of ways in which telemedicine is given moral direction. Codes of professional ethics have evolved within almost every health-care profession, framed in such a way that they bear a very close resemblance to the fundamental legal obligations incumbent on that profession: not harming others (non-maleficence) and respecting in their autonomy and privacy. Government guidelines and public policy, including specific regulations, are also of importance

Table 11.1 Legal and ethical issues in telemedicine

Issue	Content
Issues that are fundamental to telemedicine	
Ethical fundamentals	Autonomy and consent, confidentiality and other aspects of the patient–professional relationship, non-maleficence and beneficence, justice and access
Political fundamentals	National and cross-border reimbursement of patients and professionals, national programmes and strategies, funding and political direction
Issues mostly affecting the use of telemedicine	
Using and sharing health information	Consent to information sharing, confidentiality, privacy and data protection, information security management
Responsibility, liability and good practice	Duty of care, registration and training, indemnity insurance, clinical governance and risk management
Guidelines, protocols and best practice	Evolution, provenance and content of published guidelines, standards and protocols
Cross-border practice	Registration and licensure, indemnity insurance, jurisdiction and choice of law, mobility of patients and professionals, health in the EU internal market
Issues mostly affecting the supply of telemedicine	
Supplying telemedicine services	Directives on Electronic Commerce and Distance Selling, advertising of medical and pharmaceutical products, media and broadcasting regulations
Standards and interoperability	'New Approach' Directives, standards bodies, obligations relating to procurement by public bodies
Medical devices, product liability and safety	Medical devices regulations, CE marking, FDA approval, Directives on Product Liability and General Product Safety
Intellectual property rights	Copyright, patents, trademarks, design rights, passing off and other infringements, exploitation

in giving health-care a moral direction, because morality is a vital ingredient of good policy.

Political fundamentals

Regional and national governments in Western countries are being driven to provide better and more effective health care for their citizens and much of this demand has its origins in the capabilities offered by medical and surgical advances, the factors associated with democracy and, of course, the possibilities offered by information and communication technologies. Among the commonly acknowledged driving factors behind investment in telemedicine are:

- pressure to secure more acceptable levels of patient safety – telemedicine applications are acknowledged as having a key role to play in risk management and reduction (e.g. using decision support software to reduce medication errors);
- citizens and patients becoming more consumer-focused in their relationship with health-care systems and professionals – leading to the introduction of new

concepts such as choice, a demand for the best care available and intolerance of inequality of access based on geographical location (so-called 'postcode lotteries');
- the need for radical improvements in service productivity despite limited budgets – especially in countries where a significant proportion of health-care delivery has been state funded for many years and now suffers from the inertia commonly associated with very large institutions;
- the need to manage the increasing complexity of health-care processes – and to manage the resulting huge quantities of information.[3]

Using and sharing health information

Patients entrust health-care professionals with, or allow them to gather, sensitive information relating to their health and other matters as part of their seeking treatment. They do so in confidence and they have the legitimate expectation that health-care professionals will respect their privacy and act appropriately. In some circumstances patients may lack the competence to extend this trust, or may be unconscious, but this does not diminish the duty of confidence. It is essential, if the legal requirements are to be met and the trust of patients is to be retained, that health-care professionals providing a telemedicine service provide a *confidential* service.

Consequently, information that can identify individual patients must not be used or disclosed for purposes other than health care without the patient's explicit consent, some other legal basis or where not to do so may significantly increase risk for others. Unless there is robust justification for using information in a form that identifies an individual it should not be used in that form. In contrast, anonymized information is not confidential and may be used with relatively few constraints.

Anyone involved in providing a telemedicine service should have an understanding of their obligations in respect of health information and also achieve a standard of behaviour that builds on existing best practice.

Confidentiality
The principle of confidentiality has been at the heart of medical ethics since the time of Hippocrates and has been developed by various codes, including the International Code of Medical Ethics, which states that a doctor must preserve 'absolute confidentiality in all he knows about his patient' even after the patient's death. The UK's General Medical Council has made it clear:

Patients have the right to expect that you will not disclose any personal information which you learn during the course of your professional duties, unless they give permission. Without assurances about confidentiality, patients may be reluctant to give doctors the information they need in order to provide good care.[4]

In addition to a clear ethical duty to preserve patient confidentiality, there is also a legal duty of confidentiality that has evolved, in the UK for instance, out of the fields of contract, equity and property law. The overwhelming ethical duty to respect a patient's confidentiality must be balanced against the danger of maintaining silence.

Consent

It is always possible for a health-care professional to disclose confidential information where the patient gives consent. Every competent adult has an inviolable right of autonomy and self-governance – the right to determine what is done to his or her own body. Failure to obtain consent to medical treatment and to the use of information about patients is a tort and crime. The right to consent to medical treatment is offset by an accompanying right to refuse it – indeed, the possibility of a person positively refusing to consent to medical treatment, rather than simply failing to give a valid consent, must always be considered.

For consent to be valid, patients must be aware of what options are available and have the ability to make an informed choice. This therefore means that they should be given as much information as they want or need. How much or how little is adequate will vary from person to person. The UK General Medical Council's guidelines[5] state that doctors:

> must give patients the information they ask for or need about their condition, its treatment and prognosis; give information to patients in a way they can understand; [and] respect the right of patients to be fully involved in discussions about care.

Valid consent may be implicit or explicit, oral or written. In practice, consent is often assumed by the opening of the mouth for an examination of the throat, or the offering of an arm for taking blood pressure. However, assumed consent will apply only to the procedure in question.

Consent to the use of information may be assumed when patients give a health-care professional information about themselves. That is, the information will be used for the direct provision of treatment. The use of that information for research purposes very likely goes beyond what is anticipated by the average patient, and so express consent should be sought to use patient information for such purposes.

European Data Protection Directive

The European Union's Directive on Data Protection (95/46/EC) has created a harmonized regulatory regime for the privacy and security of health information throughout the member states.[6] It lays down data protection principles which must be complied with in relation to all personal data. According to the principles, health information must be processed fairly and lawfully. It must be collected for specified, legitimate purposes and not further processed in a way that is incompatible with those purposes. Where necessary, the information must be kept up to date and stored in a form that permits identification of the patient for no longer than is necessary.

European Convention on Human Rights

It used to be said that there was no general right to privacy. Whether or not this has now changed with the enactment of the European Convention on Human Rights is debateable. Article 8 of the Convention – the right to respect for private and family life – is, like the common law of confidentiality, qualified by exceptions. In the case of the Convention, the exceptions operate 'as is necessary in a democratic society in the interests of the protection of health or morals, the protection of the rights and freedoms of others and the prevention of disorder or crime'. The courts are thus required to balance the right to privacy and other important rights, such as the right to life (contained in Article 2 of the Convention), the right to freedom from torture or degrading treatment (Article 3) or the right to freedom of expression (Article 10).

Responsibility, liability and good practice

In the UK, the Bolam test[7] states that a health-care professional will not be guilty of malpractice where he or she has acted in accordance with a practice accepted as proper by a responsible body of professionals, skilled in that particular art, provided reasonable skill and care have been used. Hence a health-care professional will not have been negligent if he or she acted in accordance with a standard of practice accepted by a group of health-care professionals practising in the same specialty, notwithstanding that the group is numerically small and that a contrary body of opinion exists, provided that the standard can withstand logical analysis.

Hence malpractice – as applied to all the actions a health-care professional may undertake, including the warning of risks, obtaining of valid consent, diagnosis and selection of appropriate treatment – is judged by reference to the existence of a legal duty and the acceptable standards of practice that must be met. But given that professional standards and guidelines for telemedicine are still in their infancy, how do we decide what the 'standard of care' in telemedicine is?

First, we must ask whether or not it is standard practice to use telemedicine *at all* in the field in question. While radiology, dermatology and pathology already employ telemedicine on a regular basis, its take-up in certain other branches of medicine has been much slower. The 'four principles' approach of Beauchamp and Childress[8] includes respect for justice in the allocation of medical resources as one of the fundamental ethical principles of medical practice. But converting a perceived moral obligation – to achieve equity in health resource allocation – into a legal duty not to deny patients access to the highest standard of medical care simply by virtue of their geographical isolation is a difficult task. There have been several medical and health law cases over the past decade where courts have been reluctant to infer negligence on the part of a doctor when they felt that the real cause of harm to a patient was the failure by a hospital or health authority to allocate funds to a much needed service.[9] Although there is a growing lack of tolerance of the practice of distorting the existing law so as to conceal the real social and moral issues which arise from funding decisions, questions of health-care policy are, strictly speaking, for governments and not the courts. Hence successfully winning damages on the grounds of a health-care professional's or organization's failure to provide a telemedicine service would require such services to have become ubiquitous enough to constitute standard practice, and this is still, arguably, some way in the future.

Our second question, then, must be: if we are using telemedicine systems, what are the appropriate clinical standards or guidelines we should adopt? No one can disagree that the issue of standards must be addressed by rigorous risk assessment, backed by a high level of commitment to training and the development of proper guidelines and protocols. Providing a minimum standard of care maximizes good outcomes for patients. But movement towards adopting such standards has so far been slow.

Guidelines, protocols and best practice

Definitive guidelines have not yet been produced for telemedicine. Nonetheless, the existence of guidelines in a clinical specialty:

> can be regarded as signs of maturity in a medical technique and their absence confirms the newness or immaturity of telemedicine.[10]

It is certainly the case that few, if any, of the usual activities associated with good medical practice in countries such as the UK – for example quality assurance activities, clinical governance, professional self-regulation – have been focused specifically on the use of information and communication technologies in health and social care. One reason for this, perhaps, is that there is still insufficient published scientific evidence to support their use. Likewise, most of the professional and regulatory bodies have yet to produce specific guidance on good professional practice when using telemedicine. The Royal College of Radiologists is a notable exception.

Existing guidelines have mainly been produced by national colleges or associations of medical professionals from specific clinical specialties such as radiology, dermatology and psychiatry. Occasionally, associations such as the American Telemedicine Association (ATA) or the Internet Healthcare Coalition (IHC) have produced guidelines on specific clinical applications.

The role of guidelines in court has been summarized as follows:

> Guidelines could be introduced to a court by an expert witness as evidence of accepted and customary standards of care, but they cannot be introduced as a substitute for expert testimony. Courts are unlikely to adopt standards of care advocated in clinical guidelines as legal 'gold standards' because the mere fact that a guideline exists does not of itself establish that compliance with it is reasonable in the circumstances, or that non-compliance is negligent.[11]

Cross-border practice

Telemedicine allows the transmission of health information across the borders of nation states. Cross-border telemedicine services have begun, particularly in specialties such as teleradiology, where remote reporting centres have been established in places such as Minneapolis in the USA,[12] Leuven in Belgium[13] and Barcelona in Spain.[14] For services such as these, which deliver health care across the borders of nation states, two crucial questions must be answered:

(1) How do we decide which country's law applies and which court has jurisdiction over the service?
(2) What are the consequences of the existing system of registration and supervision for health-care professionals involved in the delivery of tele-medicine services across borders?

Jurisdiction and choice of law

The legal principles on which the applicable law and jurisdiction in cross-border transactions are based were established a long time before the invention of computers and information networks. These principles have always been used to *localize* a transaction within the jurisdiction with which it is deemed to have the closest relationship and to give that jurisdiction legal authority over the transaction. This is encapsulated in the principle that a legal action should be brought in the jurisdiction that is the most convenient and fair for all the parties concerned (*forum non conveniens*). In most cases this is based on the physical location where the people were situated when they performed the relevant act. In the case of a 'legal' person such as a company, the location of their relevant branch, registered office or trading office is usually used to decide on the relevant jurisdiction.

A contract will usually state the applicable law and jurisdiction that have been agreed by the parties, although if one of the parties is dealing as a consumer (that is to say, outside of the carrying on of their trade or profession) then different rules may apply in order to protect them. In tortious claims jurisdiction is decided on the basis of the place where harm occurred as a result of the tort (that is to say, a result of a negligent act or failure to act). The applicable law will normally be the law of the jurisdiction in which the tort was committed.[15] In other cases the applicable law and jurisdiction can be decided on the basis of factors such as the habitual place of residence or business of the person whose performance under a contract is at issue, the place where performance under the contract is to take place, the place where the contract was entered into or agreed, the place where an advertisement or invitation to enter into the contract was received or the place where a branch, agency or other establishment is situated.[16]

Professional registration and regulation

Health-care professionals in the US are registered and regulated on a state rather than on a national basis. The growth of state-to-state telemedicine services has necessitated the introduction of new laws allowing 'out-of-state' health-care professionals to treat and advise patients within a state. In most cases state legislatures have decided that health-care professionals are 'travelling' *to* the patient when they deliver health care virtually (and therefore require a licence to practise in the state) rather than considering the patient as travelling to the health-care professional. Different states have adopted different approaches, and while some (such as Kansas) will grant 'special licences' or exemptions to appropriately qualified out-of-state physicians, many will not. In those states that do not recognize out-of-state licences, such as Arizona and New Mexico, full registration within the state is still necessary. This restrictive policy also describes the situation in the European Union.

Health-care professionals who have trained and qualified in one member state of the European Union are entitled to have their qualifications recognized in all other member states. This is true not only of doctors but also of many other health-care professionals, including nurses, midwives, dentists, pharmacists, physiotherapists, occupational therapists, clinical psychologists, radiographers, optometrists and opticians. Some of these professionals are covered under what are called 'sectoral' directives, which apply to individual professions such as medicine, dentistry and pharmacy. Others are known as 'general system' directives. This latter category usually applies to professional qualifications involving three years or more of higher training. The directives in both categories have been amended over the years, most recently in 2001.[17] The European Commission has recently published a proposal to amend and amalgamate them all.[18]

The barriers and problems in this existing system as regards the migration of health professionals are also challenges for the provision of telemedicine services across borders. These include:

- The lack of any formal mechanism through which information about disciplinary procedures or criminal charges brought against a health-care professional in one member state can be shared or exchanged with the competent authorities of other member states in which that health-care professional is registered to practise.
- Significant variations between the structure and duration of specialist and general practitioner training found in the different member states.
- Significant variations between the member states in their requirements for continuing medical education. While most health-care professionals would tend to agree that professional development is, at the very least, an ethical obligation, the extent to which it is a legal obligation varies from country to country.

- Inadequate language skills, which are undoubtedly a practical barrier to safe medical practice, as well as cultural differences which make it difficult for health-care professionals in one member state to understand how health services are delivered in another member state.
- Differences of approach between member states as regards malpractice liability insurance. Most liability insurers do not permit an insured person to practise outside their country of registration.
- Difficulties in obtaining reimbursement from a national health system or statutory insurance scheme for the costs of treatment delivered using a tele-medicine service.

Supplying telemedicine services

The European Commission believes that telemedicine is part of an emerging industry which

> has the potential to be the third largest industry in the health sector with a turnover of €11 billion. By 2010 it could account for 5% of the total health budget.

What are the laws and regulations that will govern the way in which that business will be conducted? There are three important European Union Directives.

Distance selling

The European Union's Directive on distance selling (1997/7/EC) covers all forms of distance selling, not just that which takes place over the Internet. It provides for a very wide definition of a 'distance contract'. The Directive requires that the promotional techniques used in distance selling must pay due regard to the consumer's privacy and that two particular forms of communication – automated calling systems and fax machines – cannot be used without the prior consent of the consumer. Arguably then, the sending of unsolicited emails (a practice known as 'spamming') should also be subject to consent.

Telemedicine suppliers who send unsolicited commercial emails therefore need to be aware that, while the practice is not illegal in the UK and other European countries (with the exception of Austria, which has banned the practice), they need to make frequent reference to lists such as the Direct Marketing Association's voluntary email preference service (similar to the telephone and mailing preference systems already established) and give the recipient of their emails a clear means of opting out of receiving further messages from them.

In terms of the formation of an online contract, the Directive on distance selling requires that certain information must be provided by the supplier to the consumer. This includes the identity of the vendor, the nature and cost of the goods and services that are to be supplied and the delivery arrangements. This information must be supplied in written or other appropriate form. A confirmatory email would appear to be sufficient for this purpose.

Electronic commerce

The European Union's Directive on legal aspects of electronic commerce (2000/31/EC) applies to any service normally provided for remuneration, at a distance, by electronic means and at the individual request of a recipient of services. The Directive makes a number of provisions relating to the law governing electronic contracts and how those contracts are formed. It also provides that any contract entered into by electronic means should be governed by the law of the place in which the supplier is established. This provision, however, is in direct conflict with the provisions contained in the Brussels and Rome Conventions, which state that all consumer contracts are subject to the law of the country where the consumer lives. It is unclear which provisions should be given primacy but, in any event, the Directive tries to prevent disputes that might arise in electronic contracts from proceeding to the stage of litigation by requiring both member states and the European Commission to draw up, at Community level, codes of conduct 'designed to contribute to the implementation of the substantive provisions of the Directive'. This requires, among other things, the creation of 'out-of-court' schemes for dispute resolution, including appropriate electronic means.

The nature of the Internet is such that in forming a contract with another party it may be necessary to use one or more Internet service providers or a portal that directs Internet users to a number of services. The Directive on electronic commerce contains provisions intended to limit or exclude the liability of these so-called 'intermediaries' where they are acting as 'mere conduits' for transmissions sent and received by third parties.

Electronic signatures

The European Union's Directive on electronic signatures (1999/93/EC) was given final approval in December 1999 and member states were given until 19 July 2001 to implement the measure. The Directive's main purpose is to encourage the development of electronic equivalents to written documents and manual signatures in a technologically neutral manner (i.e. in a way that does not refer to any specific system for electronic signatures, such as public key encryption). Two forms of signatures are identified in the Directive: 'electronic' and 'advanced'. An 'electronic' signature is information in electronic form which is either attached to or logically associated with other electronic information and which serves as a method of identification. An 'advanced' signature means an electronic signature that meets four specific criteria set out in Article 2(1) of the Directive. Such 'advanced' signatures require the use of some form of encryption and are given the same status in relation to electronic information as a handwritten signature has in relation to paper-based data. This means, for instance, that they are admissible as evidence in legal proceedings provided that they have been certified by an independent agency (a so-called 'certification service provider') acting as a trusted third party. Almost anyone can set themselves up as a trusted third party, issuing certified advanced electronic signatures, although the Directive provides that:

Member States may introduce or maintain voluntary accreditation schemes aiming at enhanced levels of certification-service provision. All conditions related to such schemes must be objective, transparent, proportionate and non-discriminatory. Member States may not limit the number of accredited certification-service-providers for reasons which fall within the scope of this Directive.

Standards and interoperability

Telemedicine is a field with differing technical standards, such as for communication between systems and networks, for the recording and sharing of electronic patient information and for the protection of the security, integrity and authenticity of electronically stored and transmitted data. One reason for the lack of agreement on standards is that the field of health information is complex. The rapidly evolving technology is another factor, demanding that standards be developed for a diverse range of applications. The sectors that have grown the fastest are those in which there are open, published standards and technical specifications, for instance HL7 for data transmission and DICOM for image transmission.

Most of these technical standards are not 'legal standards' as such. That is to say, they are not legally binding by virtue merely of their existence. Occasionally, their application can become a legal requirement where this is explicitly provided for in a legislative instrument. It is much more common, however, for the adoption of a particular technical standard to be one of a number of ways in which an individual or organization can comply with the law. In most cases, therefore, standards may enable compliance with the law but their use is not, *de facto*, a legal necessity.

Under the Council Decision (87/95/EEC) of 22 December 1986 on standardization in the field of information technology and telecommunications, the institutions of the European Union are obliged to take measures to facilitate the promotion and application of standards in public sector orders and procurement, and in technical regulations.

Medical devices, product liability and safety

Telemedicine requires the transmission of health information from one place to another. From a legal point of view, the quality of the information on which a health professional bases an opinion or diagnosis raises an important question about the division of responsibility between the health-care professional and the provider of the telemedicine service. It is important for health-care professionals using such a service to recognize, for instance, when clinical information is and is not of appropriate quality to make a diagnosis.

Consider teleradiology. A missed diagnosis might occur because of negligence on the part of the distant radiologist. However, if a diagnosis was missed because of a technical failure in the telemedicine service with which the X-ray image was sent, then one or more of the organizations involved in the provision of the service may be liable. In addition, other parties may be considered to be negligent, including the manufacturer or supplier of:

- the X-ray equipment and/or any of its components, including software, with which the image was captured and transmitted;
- the telecommunications network over which the images were sent;
- the equipment with which the image was received and viewed by the consultant radiologist and any of its components, including software.

Moreover, any individual or organization involved in the inspection, maintenance, repair or upgrade of any of the above elements of a telemedicine service may also be potentially liable for the failure of the service. So while the term 'product' liability may *sound* as though it provides for responsibilities on the part only of the producer of a telemedicine product, in fact any individual or organization involved in the service has responsibilities and may face potential liability. Problems can arise, however, where one or more of those parties is insolvent, uninsured or unidentifiable. Moreover, there may be further difficulties if one or more parties are located in different jurisdictions.

Medical devices

Since 14 June 1998 all medical devices must comply with the European Union's Directive concerning medical devices (93/42/EEC), under which medical devices must comply with the essential requirements of the Directive and obtain a 'CE mark' as evidence of compliance before being marketed. The definition of a 'medical device' is:

> any instrument, apparatus, appliance, material or other article, whether used alone or in combination, including the software necessary for its proper application intended by the manufacturer to be used for human beings for the purpose of:
>> diagnosis, prevention, monitoring, treatment or alleviation of disease,
>> diagnosis, monitoring, treatment, alleviation of or compensation for an injury or handicap,
>> investigation, replacement or modification of the anatomy or of a physiological process,
>> control of conception,
> and which does not achieve its principal intended action in or on the human body by pharmacological, immunological or metabolic means, but which may be assisted in its function by such means.[19]

Manufacturers of medical devices are obliged to ensure that these essential requirements are met in relation to each product. A competent authority in each member state of the European Union is expected to implement the requirements of the Directive, to ensure compliance, to evaluate adverse incidents and to carry out assessments of devices intended for clinical investigation. The UK competent authority is the Medicines and Health-care products Regulatory Agency (MHRA). Among the services provided by competent authorities such as the MHRA is a system for reporting adverse incidents involving medical devices, under which manufacturers are required to report adverse incidents to the Agency immediately on hearing about them, even where user error rather than a device problem is suspected.

The European Council Directive concerning medical devices provides for a broadly similar regulatory regime to that enforced by the Food and Drug Administration (FDA) in the US.

Product liability

Product liability is used to describe the civil liability – as opposed to criminal liability – of manufacturers and others for any harm caused by the defective condition of a product. There are, broadly speaking, three civil legal routes by which a person harmed by a defective product can seek redress, as well as some criminal penalties which may be enforced where a product fails to comply with a specified standard of safety. The first and most important route is the strict liability regime provided for under the European Union's Directive concerning liability for defective products (85/374/EEC). The second route is through contract law and the third is through the tortious law of negligence. Criminal sanctions are provided for by the European Union's Directive on general product safety (92/59/EEC).

(1) Contractual liability

Modern product liability law has partly evolved out of contract law and, in particular, out of the warranties and conditions as to the description, fitness for purpose and satisfactory quality of a product that would usually be contained in a contract for the sale or supply of goods.[20] The European Union's Directive on unfair terms in consumer contracts (93/13/EEC) provides that unfair terms used in a contract with a consumer will not be binding on the consumer. So these warranties and conditions cannot be excluded from a contract with a consumer, although they can be enforced in a business-to-business contract only if they are reasonable. More generally, a party to a contract for the sale or supply of goods cannot exclude or restrict liability for death or personal injury caused by negligence.

However, contract law has only very limited usefulness for most people who are harmed by a defective product because contract law provides a remedy only where there is a contract between the provider of the product and the buyer. In most modern health systems under which care is provided free at the point of need (i.e. in a national health system) or is reimbursed by a third party (i.e. under a statutory insurance scheme) a patient will *not* be in a contractual relationship with the provider of a health-care product. The product will have been supplied for their benefit, but it will not have been purchased directly by them. A contractual relationship will usually exist only where the health-care product is supplied privately and paid for directly by the patient or where the contract is for the supply or sale or goods or services of a type which it is usual for one person to purchase on behalf of both himself or herself and others.[21]

Where services, as opposed to goods, are sold or supplied, warranties and conditions will be implied in the contract that require the supplier to carry out the service with reasonable care and skill, within a reasonable time and to charge a reasonable price for the services rendered. These provisions have been used successfully by, for instance, the customers of software companies that provided faulty software. Even where a supplier of goods or services seeks to limit their liability for breach of contact by means of a limitation clause contained in the contract itself, that clause must be 'fair and reasonable'.

(2) Tortious liability

Of much greater practical usefulness than contract law is the tort of negligence, under which a person who is harmed by a defective product may make a claim for compensation against the producer of the defective product whose negligent act or omission to act has caused them harm. No direct contractual relationship between the person harmed and the producer of the product is required.

The duty of care owed by a manufacturer has since been extended to everyone in the service chain. So in the case of a videoconsultation between a health professional and a patient which takes place as part of a telemedicine service this duty of care could apply to many parties, including:

- the manufacturer of the videoconferencing system;
- the producer of the software that operates that system;
- the reseller that supplies the system to a user;
- the manufacturer or supplier of any middleware;
- the provider of the telecommunication network(s) used by the service;
- the provider of any telecommunication equipment used by the service;
- the health-care service provider (e.g. a hospital) that uses the system in the provision of a telemedicine service;
- the service company(s) that maintain, repair or inspect any of the above equipment.

This list is not exhaustive. Each party must exercise such care as is reasonable in all aspects of the process under their control. Their liability may arise from taking insufficient care in things like research, development and design, manufacture, presentation, instructions and training for use, and warnings about risks. Moreover, a producer's duty of care does not end when health-care products are sold. There is a continuing duty incumbent on the manufacturer and suppliers of such products to take reasonable steps to warn users about anything which might result in injury to them and to operate an appropriate system for recalling faulty products.

(3) European Directive on liability for defective products

The European Union's Directive concerning liability for defective products (85/374/EEC) was enacted, at least in part, in response to the terrible birth defects caused by the drug thalidomide in the 1960s and 1970s. It was also intended to prevent competitive distortions in the EU's internal market being caused by differences in the protection given to consumers under national laws. Under the Directive, producers are liable for damage caused by a defect in their products.[22] A 'producer' is very broadly defined as the manufacturer of a finished product, the producer of any raw material or the manufacturer of a component part and any person who, by putting his name, trademark or other distinguishing feature on the product presents himself as its producer. It also includes anyone who first places a product on the market within the EU. Hence if a 'producer' cannot be identified then a hospital, a service-providing company or an individual health professional might all find themselves liable for the harm caused by a defective product they are using in the treatment of a patient, notwithstanding that they had no role in its manufacture or distribution. This is potentially a harsh and indiscriminate legal measure for the unsuspecting provider of a telemedicine service, who will have to ensure that they keep excellent records of where they obtain their equipment and services from, and whom they deal with. They will also need to obtain insurance and indemnities against insolvency and liability, as appropriate.

Liability under the Directive is 'strict' in the sense that there is no need to prove that the producer of the product was negligent. All the injured person has to prove is that the product was defective, that they have been harmed by the product and that there was a causal relationship between the defect and the damage. That damage includes death, personal injury and damage to or loss of property. Where two or more persons are liable for the same harm, they are held to be jointly and severally liable.

Intellectual property rights

Intellectual property is knowledge or expertise that is capable of being owned, usually by a legal person such as a company or other organization, but often by a natural person – that is to say, an individual. The different forms of intellectual property right confer rights on their owners to exploit an innovative idea or process that they have created and to benefit from doing so. The main types of intellectual property rights that will be of relevance to the suppliers of telemedicine are:

(1) *Copyright law.* Software and databases may be protected by copyright law that protects a work against unauthorized copying for the lifetime of the author plus an additional period of 70 years after their death. Protection is provided under the Berne Convention and the Directive on the harmonization of certain aspects of copyright and related rights in the information society (2001/21/EC) as well as the Directive on the legal protection of computer

programs (91/250/EEC) and the Directive on the legal protection of databases (1996/9/EC).

(2) *Patents.* The European Patent Convention provides for a single system of patent registration and protection for technologies that demonstrate the required level of novelty, inventiveness and a capacity for industrial application. Protection lasts for four years and may be renewed annually for up to 20 years.

(3) *Trademarks.* Trademarks relating to telemedicine technologies or services, consisting of words, designs, letters or numerals, may be protected under the Directive to approximate the laws of the member states relating to trademarks (89/104/EEC). Once registered they are protected indefinitely.

(4) *Design rights.* These automatically subsist in an original design and protect the outward shape and appearance of an article.

(5) *Registered design.* This is a monopoly right for the outward appearance of an article or a set of articles that lasts for a maximum of 25 years. A registered design is additional to any design right or copyright protection that may exist automatically in the design.

Conclusion

There are many questions about the legal and ethical aspects of telemedicine generally, and by and large they remain to be answered definitively. Health-care professionals who undertake telemedicine should act in a prudent manner to minimize the possibility of medicolegal complications.[23]

References

1   Brahams D. The medico-legal implications of teleconsulting in the UK. *J Telemed Telecare* 1995;**1**:196–201

2   Western Governors' Association Telemedicine Action Report. See http://www.health.state.nd.us/ndhd/pubs/tech/telemed.htm (last checked 20 August 2005)

3   Commission of the European Communities. Communication from the Commission to the Council, the European Parliament, the European Economic and Social Committee and the Committee of the Regions. Modernising social protection for the development of high-quality, accessible and sustainable health care and long-term care: support for the national strategies using the 'open method of communication'. COM(2004) 304 final. Brussels, 20 April 2004

4   General Medical Council. *Duties of a Doctor – Confidentiality: Guidance from the General Medical Council.* London: GMC, 1995

5   General Medical Council. *The Duties of a Doctor: Guidance from the General Medical Council.* London: GMC, 1995

6   Directive 95/46/EC of the European Parliament and of the Council of 24 October 1995 on the protection of individuals with regard to the processing of personal data and on the free movement of such data

7   Bolam v. Friern Hospital Management Committee [1957] 1 WLR 582 at p. 586

8   Beauchamp TL, Childress JF. *Principles of Biomedical Ethics.* 4th edn. New York: Oxford University Press, 1994

9   See, for instance, Cruisey v. St Helier NHS Trust (unreported)

10 Loane M, Wootton R. A review of guidelines and standards for telemedicine. *J Telemed Telecare* 2002;**8**:63–71

11   Hurwitz B. *Clinical Guidelines and the Law: Negligence, Discretion and Judgment*. Oxon: Radcliffe Medical Press, 1998

12   *Virtual Radiologic*. See http://www.virtualrad.net (last checked 20 August 2005)

13   *Eurorad*. See http://www.eurorad.com (last checked 20 August 2005)

14   *Telemedicine Clinic*. See http://www.telemedicineclinic.com (last checked 20 August 2005)

15   Article 5(3) of the Rome Convention on the Law Applicable to Contractual Obligations and Article of the European Communities Convention on Jurisdiction and Enforcement of Judgements in Civil and Commercial Matters (also known as the Brussels Convention)

16   Article 4(2) of the Rome Convention and Articles 5(1), 5(5), 13(3)(a) and 13(3)(b) of the Brussels Convention

17   Directive 2001/19/EC of the European Parliament and of the Council of 14 May 2001 amending Council Directives 89/48/EEC and 92/51/EEC on the general system for the recognition of professional qualifications and Council Directives 767/452/EEC, 77/453/EEC, 78/686/EEC, 78/687/EEC, 78/1026/EEC, 78/1027/EEC, 80/154/EEC, 80/154/EEC, 80/155/EEC, 85/384/EEC, 85/432/EEC, 85/433/EEC and 93/16/EEC concerning the professions of nurse responsible for general care, dental practitioner, veterinary surgeon, midwife, architect, pharmacist and doctor

18   Proposal for a Directive on the recognition of professional qualifications (COM(2002) 119)

19   Article 1(2) of Council Directive 93/42/EEC of 14 June 1993 concerning medical devices

20   In the UK, for instance, see sections 13(1) and 14(2) of the Sale of Goods Act 1979 as amended by section 1 of the Sale and Supply of Goods Act 1994

21   Such as a family holiday in the case of *Jackson* v. *Horizon Holidays* Ltd [1975] 1 WLR 1468 (CA)

22   Council Directive 85/374/EEC of 25 July 1985 on the approximation of the laws, regulations and administrative provisions of the member states concerning liability for defective products

23   Stanberry B. The legal and ethical aspects of telemedicine. 1: Confidentiality and the patient's rights of access. *J Telemed Telecare* 1997;**3**:179–87 (and three other parts)

▶12

Sources of information on telemedicine

Nancy A Brown

Introduction

In the first edition of this book, published in 1999, I began this chapter with the following:

> If we required a few words to characterize the late 1990s – the so-called 'Information Age' – a quotation from John Naisbitt's *MegaTrends* might suffice: 'We are drowning in information but starved for knowledge.'[1] With the advent of world-wide use of fax machines, cell phones, pagers, satellite communications and the Internet, we can choose to be bombarded with a continuous stream of information from anywhere in the world. The 1991 Persian Gulf War, the war we all watched from our living rooms, must be regarded as a turning point in how the public has come to accept and demand this instant access to world-wide events. There is a danger inherent in this bombardment, however. As Naisbitt has suggested, it seems that the quantity of the information or the speed with which it can be transmitted, has become valued over its quality, usefulness or credibility.

The continued growth of the Web over the past six years has not changed this situation. We are still 'drowning in information', and with the advent since 1999 of personal digital assistants (PDAs), mobile phones with Internet access, and wireless Internet access in airports and cafes, the deluge has become almost a tidal wave. Not only has the quantity of information increased hugely, we now have a wide variety of methods with which to access it. This makes it easier, for instance, to connect with friends and family from anywhere in the world, to take photographs and send them rapidly via computer or mobile phone, to download music with mobile phones and for health professionals to access medical records instantly at the bedside. But for those of us who still plod through the Web with our PC looking for information on a specific subject such as telemedicine, have things got better? Have the quality and specificity of information retrieved improved at all? More to the point, have we found what we were looking for?

Information and telemedicine

Except for possibly teleradiology, which is widely practised around the world, telemedicine is still viewed as outside the mainstream of most health-care services. It does not appear that there has been a decrease in the number of telemedicine start-ups, however, and several programmes existing in 1999 were still providing services in 2004.[2] Unfortunately, many of the barriers existing in 1999 are depressingly familiar, at least in the USA. Licensure of physicians across state lines, reimbursement from Medicare and third-party payers, and malpractice insurance are still barriers to the acceptance of telemedicine, as well as to its sustainability after government grants expire. Telecommunication is also an issue, particularly in rural areas that still do not have high-bandwidth connections.

Telemedicine practitioners must keep up with the practice issues raised above, and also with the continually accelerating changes in technology. While still not standardized across various platforms, most telemedicine technology is generally easier to use and less expensive than it was in 1999. There is specialized technology for store-and-forward applications as well as for interactive telemedicine, for which there are room-based, desktop and roll-about systems (see Chapter 2). There are technologies optimized for home care and telemonitoring, mobile care and telemetry. There are numerous peripheral devices, such as stethoscopes, otoscopes and dermascopes. There are also choices to be made in the software that accompanies the hardware. To muddy the waters even further, there are numerous vendors who seem continually to be merging with each other or starting up new companies. The effort involved in keeping up with the technology alone can require hours of research.

Internet search strategies

The Internet represents a prime source of information, albeit one with the well-known problems of unregulated publishing, e.g. no peer review, no editing. The good news is that at least a few Web search engines have made it easier to retrieve and sift through information. In fact, this might now be called the 'Google Age', since, as of late 2004, no one has seriously challenged Google as the search engine of choice. Other search engines are mentioned below but it may be worthwhile to begin a discussion on searching for telemedicine information with Google, since it is the most widely used search engine in the world.

Google not only provides search results on its home page, but powers other Website search engines' results as well. More than 300 million searches a day take place on Google's servers. In May 2004, 37% of US Web surfers used Google, while Yahoo came in second with 27%.[3] MSN, AOL, Lycos and others shared the remaining 37%. Other companies, including the Microsoft Corporation, are busily trying to topple Google's domination. However, time will tell whether they will be successful.

In 1999, Basch[4] was quoted as saying that search engines in the future would become smarter and able to aggregate Web content more efficiently by utilizing a technique called 'collaborative filtering'. She was correct, as that is essentially what Google does. Google displays search results ranked by relevance to the user's search term using a proprietary algorithm based on the concept of PageRank (PageRank is a trademark). PageRank is used to measure the importance or popularity of a Web page or Website. The PageRank of a Web page is determined not only by how many other Web pages link to it, but also by the individual PageRank scores of each of those pages. Links from pages with a higher PageRank are more valuable than links from less popular pages. Through the use of PageRank, highly relevant search results are usually obtained based on what Google calls the 'collective intelligence of the Web' (echoing Basch). Paid advertisements, and attempts to manipulate a Website's position in search result ranking through techniques such as stuffing keywords in meta tags, have much less influence on the search result ranking process than they previously did.

Though much improved through Google's efforts, Web searching can still be a frustrating business. A search on 'telemedicine' on Google brings up interesting results, but also provides a cautionary tale about searching for information on the Internet. The Telemedicine Information Exchange (TIE) (http:// tie.telemed.org) Website may be used as an example of at least two interesting caveats.

One caveat is the search engine methodology itself. The TIE has long been the number one result of a Google search on 'telemedicine'. However, depending on the day, it often switches between number one and two with the *Telemedicine Today* Website, which represents a magazine that ceased publication in early 2000 (Figure 12.1). Many of the links from the homepage are broken, and the site obviously has not been updated since a short-lived revival in 2002. Although not indicated in Figure 12.1, further perusal of the sites listed on the first page of the Google results shows that only five of the first 10 sites listed are current, up-to-date sites. The other five either have not been updated in several years or, as in the case of http://www.telemedmag.com, are broken links. Number 10, the old military site http://www.matmo.org, goes to a domain page, and numbers 11 and 12 have not been updated in several years.

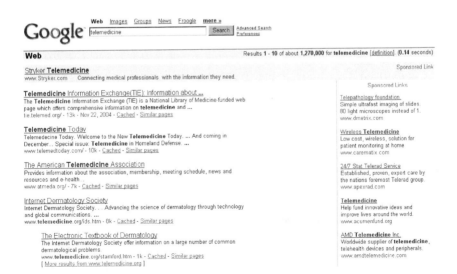

Figure 12.1 First page of results from a Google telemedicine search

The second caveat is the search term used. The continuing semantic confusion in the telemedicine community about the terms 'telemedicine' and 'telehealth' causes further problems for a search on Google. Although 'telehealth' is understood to encompass all activities associated with telecommunications technologies and health care, such as distance education, training and administration, it also encompasses the clinical applications of 'telemedicine'. However, a search on 'telehealth' on Google does not turn up several long-time telemedicine Websites. For instance, the TIE still uses the term 'telemedicine' in its title. Because of that, a search on 'telehealth' on Google will not turn up the TIE until the seventh page of results, even though the TIE arguably has more information on telehealth than any other Website on the Internet. Where it made sense, we changed several 'telemedicine' terms within the site to 'telehealth' (short of changing the name to the 'Telehealth Information Exchange'), but it made no difference. Those who do not browse past the second or third page of results will miss this valuable resource, as well as other well-established telemedicine sites that do not appear on a 'telehealth' search, such as the American Telemedicine Association (ATA) (http://www.americantelemed.org).

Advanced searches on Google using both the terms 'telemedicine' and 'telehealth' bring up another mixture of sites not found in the previous two searches, although these are basically the same sites in different orders. Google also has a 'related sites' search (click on 'similar pages' under your chosen link) which brings up a smaller set of sites related to your chosen site. As with most search engines, using fewer search terms usually provides the best results; starting with one or two words will bring the highest return, while adding terms will further narrow your search. It is also worth reading the 'Advanced Tips' sections on Google (or any other search engine) to improve the search performance.

Assiduous linking from the outdated sites mentioned above can eventually lead to valuable information, but it takes a fair amount of time and effort to determine which sites are current and which are not, leading again to 'information overload'. Of course, Google is only doing what it does well, which is to retrieve sites that are linked to by a majority of other sites. That so many out-of-date or defunct sites have still not been removed from the Web, and are still linked by credible and current sites (including, in some cases, the TIE), is evidence that Web searching is still a hit-or-miss proposition, and confirms that we are still 'drowning in information' in 2004. *Plus ça change...*

Reliable sources of telemedicine information

There is a wide variety of both electronic and print resources that have proven to be reliable sources of information. These include:

- books and reports;
- journals and trade magazines;
- the Internet (Web);
- telemedicine societies;
- conferences.

A perusal of the list of print resources from the first edition produced some surprises in 2004. Not one trade magazine from the mid-1990s has survived. *Telemedicine Today* (and its annual *Buyer's Guide*), *Telehealth Magazine*, *Telemedlaw* and *PACS and Networking News* have all ceased publication. However, the two peer-reviewed journals listed then, *Journal of Telemedicine and Telecare* (*JTT*) and *Telemedicine Journal and e-Health* (*TJ and e-Health*), are still going strong in their tenth year of existence.

The Web resources listed below are current as of late 2004. Most users are aware of the transitory nature of Websites, some of which have either disappeared completely or remain untouched since posted several years ago. A check of the posting date of any information presented is essential. The sites listed below have proven reliable through 2004 and have been continuously updated.

Books and reports

Compared with other medical subject areas, there are still relatively few print materials on the subject of telemedicine, and given the length of time it takes for most books to be published and the technology-intensive nature of telemedicine, many publications could be considered historical documents by the time they are printed. Telemedicine enjoyed a resurgence in parallel with the rise of electronic information, making much of the information about it available free or downloadable from the Web. Whether one sees that as an advantage or disadvantage may reveal individual biases. However, there are a few monographs which deserve mention as both historical documents and as basic primers on the practice and theory of telemedicine. There are also books which deal primarily with the legal aspects of telemedicine, and, unfortunately, some of those legal aspects have remained relatively unchanged since 1999. The following, with a few exceptions, are books published since 1999. A more thorough list of books, reports and conference proceedings can be found on the TIE bibliographic database (http://tie.telemed.org/biblio/) by clicking on the Browse function, or from LocatorPlus at the National Library of Medicine (http://locatorplus.gov/), which indexes books and reports.

Books
Bashshur R, Sanders JL, Shannon GW. *Telemedicine: Theory and Practice.* Springfield, IL: Charles C Thomas, 1997. 435 pp. $69.95 ISBN 0-398-0631-7
Fifteen chapters in five sections: The Context of Telemedicine; The Technology of Telemedicine; Clinical Applications of Telemedicine; Telemedicine Systems; and Telemedicine of the Future. The book also includes a glossary of terms and definitions.

Darkins AW, Cary MA. *Telemedicine and Telehealth: Principles, Policies, Performance and Pitfalls.* New York: Springer Publishing, 2000. 316 pp. $43.95 ISBN 0-8261-1302-8

Explores how the medical, social, cultural and economic dimensions associated with digital data networks will affect the kinds of health-care services we can expect to receive in future.

Frueh S, Armstrong ML. *Telecommunications for Nurses: Providing Successful Distance Education and Telehealth.* 2nd edn. New York: Springer Publishing, 2003. 304 pp. $44.95 ISBN 0-826-1984-30
Reflects the latest developments in both distance education and telehealth, focusing on practical strategies that nurses can put to use in the classroom or clinic. Each chapter is written by acknowledged experts on the particular topic.

Kinsella A. *Home Health Care: Process, Policy and Procedures.* Kensington, MD: Information for Tomorrow, 2003. 115 pp. $125.00 ISBN 0-965-7674-69
How to plan and use telehealth care to provide high-quality service in the home. Includes sample forms and policies for programme planning and development.

Maheu M, Whitten P, Allen A. *E-health, Telehealth, and Telemedicine: A Guide to Start-Up and Success.* Indianapolis: Jossey-Bass, 2001. 380 pp. $43.95 ISBN 0-787-9442-03
Primarily about the influence of communication technologies on health care. It secondarily mentions various developments in medical technology as they complete the discussion of communication technology.

Norris AC. *Essentials of Telemedicine and Telecare.* New York: John Wiley & Sons, 2001. 188 pp. $61.00 ISBN 0-471-5315-10
In a textbook for a course in health-care management, Norris (management science and information systems, University of Auckland) explains the main features of telemedicine and telecare, the potential benefits, and the limitations and barriers.

Stanberry B. *The Legal and Ethical Aspects of Telemedicine.* London: Royal Society of Medicine Press, 1998. 172 pp. £19.99 ISBN 1-85315-354-0
Examines several issues pertinent to law and telemedicine, including confidentiality, data security, malpractice, and the practice of telemedicine across state and international boundaries. Comprehensive coverage of the issues, with a European focus.

Wootton R, Batch J. *Telepediatrics and Child Health.* London: Royal Society of Medicine Press, 2004. 345 pp. £24.95 ISBN 1-85315-645-0
For all health professionals currently working or planning to set up services in paediatrics and telemedicine. This book is written by an international team of contributors who are working with paediatric telemedicine services. It covers a broad range of topics, including specialist services, primary and community services, and education.

Wootton R, Oakley A, eds. *Teledermatology*. London: Royal Society of Medicine Press, 2002. 331 pp. £24.95 ISBN 1-85315-507-1
Describes how telemedicine applies to dermatology. The aim is to permit those who are involved in dermatology to begin to assess how telemedicine might be applied to their working practice.

Wootton R, Yellowlees P, McLaren P. *Telepsychiatry and e-Mental Health*. London: Royal Society of Medicine Press, 2003. 368 pp. £19.50 ISBN 1-85315459-7
Describes how telemedicine applies to telepsychiatry and mental health generally. Represents the collective experience of practitioners in different parts of the world working with a wide range of telepsychiatry and related applications.

Reports
Bloch C. *University and State Telemedicine: Telemedicine, Telehealth, Informatics and Research*. Washington, DC: Bloch Consulting Group, 2005. 174 pp. $95.00. Updated annually (http://www.cbloch.com/university.htm)
In all, 214 listings, including detailed information and updated URLs listed conveniently state by state.

Bloch C. *Federal Agencies: Activities in Telehealth, Telemedicine, and Informatics*. Washington, DC: Bloch Consulting Group, 2005. 139 pp. $95.00 (http://www.cbloch.com/contents.htm)
A reference tool for finding current US Federal telemedicine, telehealth and informatics activities, particularly for tracking activity in Federal agencies. Updated annually.

Grigsby B, Brown N. *1999 ATSP Report on U.S. Telemedicine Activity*. Portland, OR: Association of Telehealth Service Providers, 1999. 128 pp. $49.00 (http://www.atsp.org)
A continuation of the 1998 report, profiling 132 active telemedicine programmes responding to a 1999 survey by the ATSP. Results of the survey suggested continued growth with activity in 48 states in over 1450 telemedicine-equipped facilities.

Grigsby B. *2004 TRC Report on U.S. Telemedicine Activity*. New Jersey: Civic Research Institute, 2004. 142 pp. $295 ISBN 1-887554-42-4
A continuation of the ATSP reports on US telemedicine activity, sponsored by the Telemedicine Research Center, Portland, OR. The report was based on surveys completed by 88 US programmes and submitted to the TIE, as well as anecdotal information on 54 non-US programmes. Average activity per network increased almost threefold from 2000. Many tables and figures.

Journals and trade magazines

There are two peer-reviewed journals on telemedicine, and one, the IEEE journal mentioned below, that is not focused on telemedicine but often includes articles on telemedicine-related subjects. Most other clinical peer-reviewed journals include occasional articles on specific tele-specialties. As mentioned above, there are very few trade magazines on telemedicine or teleradiology currently in publication, but many, such as *Health Data Management* and *Health Management Technology*, include occasional articles on telehealth.

Electronic magazines
Journal of Medical Internet Research. Vol. 1, 1999 – Quarterly. Free. ISSN 1438-8871 (http://www.jmir.org/index.htm). Peer-reviewed. Indexed by MEDLINE. Occasional telehealth articles.

Virtual Medical Worlds. 1997 – Monthly. Free. ISSN 1388-722X (http://www.hoise.com/vmw/04/articles/index.html). Focused on telehealth, international. Not peer reviewed.

Peer-reviewed journals
IEEE Transactions on Information Technology in Biomedicine. New Jersey: Institute of Electrical and Electronics Engineers, Vol. 1, 1997 – Quarterly. ISSN 1089-7771 (http://www.vtt.fi/tte/samba/projects/titb/titb_information/scope.html)

Journal of Telemedicine and Telecare. London: Royal Society of Medicine Press, Vol. 1, 1995 – Eight issues per year. £105 (individual), £179 (institution). ISSN 1357-633X (http://www.rsmpress.co.uk/jtt.htm)

Telemedicine Journal and e-Health. New York: Mary Ann Liebert Publishers, Vol. 1, 1995 – Six issues per year. $541 (USA), $661 (rest of world). ISSN 1078-3024 (http://www.liebertpub.com/)

Web resources

There are a number of excellent Websites offering information on telemedicine that can be recommended. The sites listed below provide a good start for any searcher, either because they offer a wide range of information or because they provide an exhaustive list of other sites to visit. They can be used as a springboard to many other good sites sponsored by specific programmes, vendors and government agencies worldwide that are well worth visiting.

Bibliographic databases
Google Scholar: http://scholar.google.com/
Google Scholar enables you to search specifically for scholarly literature, including peer-reviewed papers, theses, books, preprints, abstracts and technical

reports from all broad areas of research. It can be used to find articles from a wide variety of academic sources. Search results may include citations of older works and seminal articles that appear only in books or other offline publications. It also provides a link to those who have cited a particular article.

PubMed – The National Library of Medicine's free MEDLINE access: http://www.ncbi.nlm.nih.gov/PubMed
PubMed is the portal to free database searching on all the medical literature indexed by the National Library of Medicine since 1966. The database includes mostly clinical peer-reviewed literature on all medical disciplines and there are subject headings for 'telemedicine', 'telepathology', 'teleradiology' and 'remote consultations'. As of late 2004, a search on 'telemedicine' produced approximately 6000 citations.

TIE bibliographic database: http://tie.telemed.org/biblio/
The TIE's bibliographic database is the largest source of telemedicine citations on the Web. The database has been in existence since 1995, and has indexed all major telemedicine periodicals and literature not indexed in other sources, including abstracts if available. It also indexes historical documents from early telemedicine projects, government reports and other ephemeral literature not normally found in online databases, as well as literature from non-health sources. As of early 2004, there were approximately 15,500 citations. A document delivery service for over 5000 citations is also available.

TIE-Europe bibliographic database: http://tie.telemed.org/europe/biblio/
The TIE-Europe bibliographic database posts all non-US citations from the TIE to create a database specifically of European citations on telemedicine/telehealth.

Education and training
British Columbia Institute of Technology: http://www.bcit.ca/health/hitm/
Previously offered in separate programmes, BCIT's courses in Health Technology Management and Health Information Systems have now been combined into a single programme, Health Informatics Technology Management (HITM).

International Centre for Distance Learning: http://www-icdl.open.ac.uk/
The International Centre for Distance Learning (ICDL) is a documentation centre specializing in collecting and disseminating information on distance education worldwide. ICDL is part of the Open University Institute of Educational Technology.

Open University Institute of Educational Technology: http://iet.open.ac.uk/index.cfm
An internationally recognized centre in the UK for the research and development of online, open and distance learning.

Telehealth/e-Health Training Program, University of Calgary: http://www.fp.ucalgary.ca/telehealth/Training_Program.htm

Prepares future telehealth researchers, evaluators, professionals and consumers by providing a spectrum of formal and informal training opportunities in the discipline of telehealth.

Telemedicine Learning Center, University of California, Davis: http://www. ucdmc. ucdavis.edu/cht/tlc/
The goal of the Center is to provide an environment where practitioners, administrators, managers and telemedicine coordinators can develop the skills and knowledge needed to enhance the quality of health care in their communities.

TeleTraining Institute: http://www.teletrain.com/
The TTI provides a practical laboratory at Stillwater, Oklahoma, where teachers, corporate trainers, government instructors and others can learn and explore the skills and methods specific to the field of distance education and videoconferencing.

US Distance Learning Association: http://www.usdla.org
A non-profit association that promotes development and applications for distance learning and training.

Equipment

Med-e-Tel Telemedicine and eHealth Directory: http://www.medetel.lu/
Med-e-Tel – in cooperation with the International Telecommunication Union (ITU) and the International Society for Telemedicine (ISfT) – have prepared a Telemedicine and eHealth Directory, which incorporates a list of manufacturers and suppliers of telemedicine, telecare and e-health-related products, services and projects. Updated annually.

Telemedicine Information Exchange (TIE) Vendors Page: http://tie.telemed.org/vendors/
The TIE provides an extensive database of international vendors of telemedicine equipment and services, searchable alphabetically by name, by location, or by type of product.

General telemedicine

Canadian eHealth Initiatives Database: http://209.217.71.106/cgi-bin/starfinder/ 0?path = hihinit.txt&id = webber&pass = ANON&OK
A database of over 70 Canadian telemedicine programmes. Enter 'telemedicine' in the keyword field.

European Health Telematics Observatory (EHTO): http://www.ehto.org/
EHTO aims to collect and disseminate the most valuable information on all relevant issues relating to health telematics, including European standards, regulatory and ethical issues. It also offers a space for displaying interactive news, and a space for online virtual electronic demonstrations; available to users, industry and service providers.

Hardin Meta-Directory, from the University of Iowa: http://www.lib.uiowa.edu/hardin/md/telemed.html
The meta-directory links to sites in all specialties of medicine which in turn include lengthy lists of sites. It includes a section on telemedicine.

MedWeb: Emory University: http://www.MedWeb.Emory.Edu/MedWeb/
A search on telemedicine produces an alphabetical list of over 100 links to telemedicine sites.

Telemedicine and E-health Information Service (TEIS): http://www.teis.nhs.uk/
The objectives of TEIS are to bring together those working in the field of telemedicine, telecare and e-health; to encourage them to share information and experience and to provide an information resource for telemedicine activity in the UK.

TIE: http://tie.telemed.org
Sponsored by the Telemedicine Research Center, Portland, Oregon. A comprehensive source of information on telemedicine, including: a bibliographic database of over 15,000 citations indexing all major telemedicine publications since 1995, with a document delivery service for over 5000 selected articles; information on over 150 major international telemedicine programmes; an international list of telemedicine meetings and conferences; vendors of telemedicine equipment; sections on home health telemedicine and legal aspects of telemedicine; an extensive list of links to other telemedicine resources and much more.

TIE-EU: http://www.tieurope.org
A European spin-off of the TIE which posts non-US information from the TIE, including bibliographic citations and details of meetings. It also includes information not found on the TIE, including a series of Tool Kits on telemedicine specialties, such as teledermatology and teleradiology.

Government agency/military telemedicine

Office for the Advancement of Telehealth: http://telehealth.hrsa.gov/welcome.htm
The US Health Resources and Services Administration (HRSA) has established the Office for the Advancement of Telehealth to serve as a leader in telehealth, a focal point for HRSA's telehealth activities and as a catalyst for the wider adoption of advanced technologies in the provision of health-care services and education. The Office for the Advancement of Telehealth also administers a telehealth grant programme.

Telemedicine and Advanced Technology Research Center: http://www.tatrc.org/
TATRC is a subordinate element of the United States Army Research and Materiel Command (USARMC), and is charged with managing core Research

Development Test and Evaluation (RDT&E) functions and congressionally mandated projects in telemedicine and advanced medical technologies.

Legal issues

Avienda: http://www.avienda. co.uk/content.html
Avienda is a company based in Wales that provides professional services and advice to organizations and individuals that are implementing, using or supplying e-health, telemedicine and other health-care technologies.

Center for Telemedicine Law (CTL): http://www.ctl.org/
CTL is a non-profit entity founded by organizations committed to providing high-quality patient services through the use of telemedicine systems throughout the US and the world.

News

eHealth Infosource Cybersante: http://www.hc-sc.gc.ca/ohih-bsi/pubs/bulletin/infosource_e.html
A resource published by the Health and the Information Highway Division, Health Canada, for news, conferences and documents on e-health worldwide.

Federal Telemedicine Update: http://www.federaltelemedicine.com/
News briefs sent out every few weeks with information from Federal agencies and Capitol Hill of interest to the telemedicine, telehealth and informatics community.

iHealthBeat: http://ihealthbeat.org/
A news page from the California Healthcare Foundation covering the various ways that the Internet affects health care, including electronic medical records, telehealth and legislation. Offers a daily news email subscription on a subject of choice.

Med-e-Tel Newsletter: http://www.medetel.lu
A comprehensive international newsletter with information on a variety of issues pertinent to telemedicine, particularly the trade industry as it relates to telemedicine and telehealth.

TIE What's New: http://tie.telemed.org/news/
The TIE news column has a subscriber base of 1650, and provides news on grant openings, new technology, international news, legislation and state news. Bi-monthly.

UKeHA – UK eHealth Association Newsletter: http://www.ukeha.org.uk/augsept04newsletter/index.html
A variety of e-health news in the UK, including association news, vendors, new technology, projects. Bimonthly.

Teleradiology
American College of Radiology (ACR): http://www.acr.org/s_acr/sec.asp?CID = 967&DID = 14712
Publishes the ACR Standard for Teleradiology, which defines the goals, qualifications of personnel, equipment guidelines, licensing, credentialing, liability, communications, quality control and quality improvement for teleradiology.

Radiological Society of North America (RSNA): http://www.rsna.com/
The mission of the RSNA is to promote and develop the highest standards of radiology and related sciences through education and research. Includes many exhibits and presentations on teleradiology at its annual RSNA conference.

Royal College of Radiologists: http://www.rcr.ac.uk/
This site contains a wide range of information on College activities and resources.

TIE Links/Teleradiology: http://tie.telemed.org/links/specialties.asp#34
An extensive set of links to teleradiology and PACS information, including meta-sites, full-text articles and teleradiology services.

Listservs
Telehealth: telehealth@maelstrom.stjohns.edu
St John's University, Jamaica, New York 11439
A professional discussion forum for all applications of telehealth. To subscribe: send mail to listserv@maelstrom.stjohns.edu with the command 'SUBSCRIBE TELEHEALTH' in the body of the message.

Telemedicine: http://listserv@jiscmail.ac.uk
University of Portsmouth, UK
Use of telemedicine in the UK. To subscribe, go to: http://www.jiscmail.ac.uk/ and complete the form.

Search engines
AltaVista: http://www.altavista.com
AltaVista is consistently rated among the top five search engines on the Web. It searches more of the Web (approximately 40%) than other search engines.

Google: http://google.com
Google is widely regarded as the best search engine on the Web. Users may set up a news alert for a specific term such as telemedicine and/or telehealth and receive daily news on those subjects. Google is characterized by hyper-fast searches, consistent relevance, a large catalogue, archived pages, spell check, toolbars, a shopping page (Froogle), an image search, google scholar and a banner-free interface. It is published in nearly 100 different languages.

Health on the Net: http://www.hon.ch/HomePage/Home-Page.html
A combined search engine and database of high-quality health information.

Yahoo: http://www.yahoo.com
Yahoo recently switched to 'automated-crawling' like Google. With the acquisition of Alltheweb, GoTo (Overture) and Altavista, Yahoo is now an amalgam of many different database technologies. It is also a consumer portal like MSN, providing shopping, news and other services.

Telemedicine societies

Table 12.1 lists the major telemedicine associations and societies worldwide. Most have been in existence for several years and some of the societies organize major

Table 12.1 Telemedicine societies

Name	Purpose	URL
American Telemedicine Association	The ATA is a non-profit-making association promoting greater access to medical care via telecommunications technology. It was established in 1993, and sponsors an annual meeting which draws over a thousand delegates interested in telemedicine.	http://americantelemed.org
Association of Telehealth Service Providers	The ATSP is a non-profit-making organization created to meet the information, management and policy needs of health-care providers that are, or expect to be, providers of telemedicine services.	http://www.atsp.org
Canadian Society of Telehealth	The CST leads the transformation of health care in Canada through information and communication technology by providing a forum for advocacy, communication and sharing of resources among communities of interest.	http://www.cst-sct.org/index.php
Danish Society for Clinical Telemedicine	The aim of the Danish Society is, based on science, to promote knowledge and understanding for the use of telemedicine and telemedical tools in clinical settings.	http://www.dskt.org/
Finnish Society of Telemedicine	The aims of the Finnish Society of Telemedicine are to promote the health of the population through telecommunication and to disperse expert knowledge within health care.	http://www.fimnet.fi
International Society for Telemedicine	The ISfT's goal is to promote the development of telemedicine, telecare and telehealth around the world. The Society acts as a forum for the exchange of information and ideas among all those interested in the telemedicine field.	http://isft.org
Telemedicine Forum of the Royal Society of Medicine	An academic (i.e. disinterested) body, with no commercial affiliations, based at the Royal Society of Medicine in London. Membership is not restricted to doctors, and the Forum actively encourages participation from industry, government, hospital management and the paramedical professions.	http://www.rsm.ac.uk
The UK eHealth Association	The UK eHealth Association (formerly the UK Telemedicine Association) has been formed to represent all those corporations and individuals interested in the development of e-health in the United Kingdom.	http://www.ukeha.org.uk/news/news_page.html

Table 12.2 Major telemedicine and telehealth conferences

Name	Purpose	URL
American Telemedicine Association Annual Meeting and Exposition	An annual conference, usually in the first half of the year, which draws over a thousand delegates interested in telemedicine. Includes a large vendor exhibition. Abstracts published in the *Telemedicine Journal and e-Health*.	http://americantelemed.org
Canadian Society of Telehealth Annual Meeting	Over 400 delegates with international speakers and an industry trade exhibition.	http://www.cst-sct.org/index.php
Congress of the International Society for Telemedicine	Sponsored by the International Society for Telemedicine (ISfT), this annual conference includes a wide variety of presentations of interest to telemedicine users worldwide.	http://isft.org
Med-e-Tel Annual Exhibition and Trade Show	Held in Luxembourg, the show focuses on the industry aspect of telemedicine with several vendor exhibits and a vendor directory, as well as presentations on research results.	http://www.medetel.lu
Medical Imaging SPIE International Symposium	Sponsored by the International Society for Optical Engineering (SPIE), this annual conference provides presentations on visualization, image-guided procedures and display; physics of medical imaging; physiology, function and structure from medical images; image processing; PACS and imaging informatics, and more.	http://spie.org/app/conferences/index.cfm
Medicine Meets Virtual Reality: MMVR	In its 13th year in 2004, this conference is designed as a forum for encouraging and sharing innovative research on information-based tools for clinical care and medical education.	http://www.nextmed.com/mmvr_virtual_reality.html
PACS Annual Conference	Sponsored by the Department of Radiology of the University of Rochester School of Medicine and Dentistry, presentations include clinical applications that emphasize PACS as a tool of the entire health-care enterprise.	http://www.urmc.rochester.edu/pacs2005/
Successes and Failures in Telehealth (SFT)	Sponsored by the Centre for Online Health at the University of Queensland, Brisbane, Australia, the SFT series has successfully been built on a theme that had not previously been attempted. The meeting provides a very open and frank forum for the presentation of both successful and not so successful telehealth initiatives. The full proceedings are published in the *Journal of Telemedicine and Telecare*.	http://www.uq.edu.au/sft/
Telemed and eHealth	An annual conference sponsored by the Telemedicine Forum of the Royal Society of Medicine, UK. The full proceedings are published in the *Journal of Telemedicine and Telecare*.	http://www.rsm.ac.uk
Tromsø Telemedicine and e-Health Conference	Organized by the Norwegian Centre for Telemedicine in collaboration with STAKES (the National Research and Development Centre for Welfare and Health, Finland), FFO (the Norwegian Federation of Organizations of Disabled People), DNK (the Norwegian Cancer Society) and FCHP (the Finish Centre of Health Promotion).	http://www.telemed.no/index.php?cat=16611

annual conferences. Benefits vary according to the size of the organization, but they all provide a valuable means of networking with others interested in telemedicine.

Telemedicine conferences

Table 12.2 lists major telemedicine conferences worldwide. Many are sponsored by the telemedicine societies mentioned above. While conference vendor exhibitions and presentations are very useful for keeping up to date with telemedicine, networking with peers worldwide is one of the major benefits of these conferences. Many other large conferences, such as those sponsored by the Health Information Management Systems Society (HIMSS, http://www.himss.org) and the Radiology Society of North America (RSNA, http://www.rsna.org), include a fair amount of telemedicine/teleradiology on their conference programme. Many meetings, for example, the Forums presented by the Royal Society of Medicine, the Telehealth Leadership Conference organized by the University of Missouri Telehealth Program and the ATA's Home Health Conference, also offer more focused subject areas for smaller numbers of attenders. A comprehensive list of conferences may be found on the TIE's Meetings page at http://tie.telemed.org/meetings/.

Conclusion

While telemedicine cannot yet be considered to be part of mainstream health care, it has become a more familiar part of health terminology worldwide. In the US, there are frequent articles about it in online news magazines and specialty journals, more mention of it by government policy analysts concerned with the adoption of technology in health-care overall, and at least some telemedicine activity at every major medical school in the country. It is still mostly ignored in medical school curriculums, although that is improving with more training in the use of computers and personal digital assistants in health care. Its use particularly seems to be thriving in home care and corrections care, as well as mental health care. In the US, there is slow but steady progress towards full Medicare reimbursement, and both the US and the UK have been mandated by their respective governments to begin extensive changes over the next 10 years to incorporate technology for electronic medical records, drug prescriptions and telemedicine.

References

1   Naisbitt J. *MegaTrends: Ten New Directions Transforming our Lives.* New York: Warner Books, 1984
2   Grigsby B. *2004 TRC Report on US Telemedicine Activity.* New Jersey: Civic Research Institute Press, 2004
3   Search Engine Watch. See http://searchenginewatch.com/reports/article.php/2156431 (last checked 12 December 2004)
4   Basch R. Information presented in a keynote speech at the Online Northwest Conference. Portland, OR, 12 February 1999

▶13

Telemedicine in the future

Paul J Heinzelmann, Nancy E Lugn and Joseph C Kvedar

Introduction

Telemedicine has survived the high expectations associated with the 'technology bubble' of the 1990s and its eventual collapse. It continues to thrive. However, forecasting the future of telemedicine is largely speculative, and varying opinions about the future of telemedicine and e-health have been expressed.[1–4]

Why telemedicine in the future?

Although life expectancy is increasing throughout the world, there is significant morbidity and mortality from chronic diseases such as heart disease, cancer and diabetes,[5] and the ageing of the population will make things worse in future. There is also evidence that high-quality and cost-effective health interventions are not being used effectively on a regional, national or global scale.[6] This results in over-use, under-use and misuse of resources, long waiting times to access medical specialists, significant practice variability and poor adherence to established standards of care.

Enormous potential exists to improve health services throughout the world by using information and communication technologies (ICTs) to expand access to primary, secondary and tertiary care, raise quality, increase efficiency and decrease costs.[7–9] The burden of chronic disease, for example, can be significantly lessened through telemonitoring to decrease emergency room visits, hospital admissions, hospital stays and costs.[10,11] Telemedicine-based disease management has also been shown to improve outcomes such as blood pressure, glucose control,[12,13] medication compliance, functional status and quality of life.[14,15]

By providing greater access to medical expertise, telemedicine can reduce the geographical variability of diagnosis and clinical management. Teleconsultation has been shown to change diagnoses and management recommendations, and also to reduce the long waiting times associated with access to high-demand specialty care.[16] This is particularly valuable in the developing world, where specialist care is often inaccessible.[17]

There are many examples of why telemedicine provides a compelling alternative to conventional acute, chronic and preventive care, and how it can improve clinical outcomes.

Who will be the future users of telemedicine?

The future users of telemedicine will be patients and providers. The spectrum of patients, however, will probably broaden to include not only ill patients, but also those recently diagnosed, those at risk for disease, the 'worried well' and health-conscious consumers. Providers will include the traditional physician and nurse, but will also include less skilled health professionals as they enter the workforce and health care takes on a broader team approach. This will also include carers, who may be family members or other non-professionals.

Where will it be used?

One advantage of telemedicine is that it depends less on location and time than traditional care. In the industrialized world, it is likely that telemedicine will continue to move health-care delivery from the hospital or clinic into the home. In some instances, health care will continue to the individual patient level. For example, heart failure patients may have their vital signs and other indicators monitored during their routine daily activities. Any readings outside a pre-determined range can be forwarded to a provider who can intervene as required.

In contrast, telemedicine in the developing world or in regions with limited infrastructure will mainly be used in applications that link providers based at health centres, referral hospitals and tertiary centres.

How will the future of telemedicine be determined?

The future of telemedicine will depend on: (1) human factors, (2) economic factors and (3) technology.

Human factors
Behaviours related to technology are influenced by our culture, knowledge, attitudes, beliefs, practices and routines. These, in turn, affect change at the individual, organizational and societal levels.

Patients
Patient behaviour and perceptions will guide telemedicine in the years ahead as patients come to appreciate and expect high-quality, technology-enabled health care. Several trends indicate that this is already happening:

- the increasing use of the Internet for health-related purposes;[18]
- growing demand for faster local access to medical services;
- growing dissatisfaction with the current health system;
- greater patient participation in health-care decision-making;

- high levels of patient satisfaction with telemedicine;[3,19]
- increasing use of the Internet and mobile phone technologies globally.

Providers

The supply of health-care providers, their perceptions and their behaviour will also be important. Significant trends include:

- anticipated shortages in physician and nursing workforces;[20,21]
- less skilled health professionals and lay carers are playing a larger role, increasing the need for communication among the various providers;
- provider adoption of e-health technologies into clinical practice is occurring, but with some resistance.[22,23]

Telemedicine services can add value by redistributing medical expertise, integrating the contributions of multidisciplinary providers and creating new educational opportunities.

Organizations

Health-care provider organizations have begun to shift their emphasis from episodic care to continuous care, as chronic disease management and prevention become part of their mission. They are also using less skilled and less costly providers as a part of a multidisciplinary approach to health-care delivery. In addition, the basis on which health-care organizations are competing is beginning to evolve from one based on cost shifting to one based on performance and quality.[24,25] Although there has been some resistance, these types of initiatives are likely to gain momentum.

In general, support for technology-enabled health care appears to be occurring within health-care provider, payer, employer and patient advocacy organizations. This support is reflected in policies and practices that encourage future use of ICTs. Such organizations include the American Association of Retired Persons (AARP), the Institute of Medicine (IOM), the National Health Service (NHS), the World Health Organization (WHO)[26] and the World Bank.

Finally, organizational adoption of new health interventions is usually accelerated by scientific evidence of their benefit. There has been an increase in the number of telemedicine clinical trials conducted over the past decade, although further work is required.[27] Figure 13.1 illustrates the number of studies identified as clinical trials through MEDLINE using the search terms 'telemedicine' and 'telehealth'.

Society

Within industrialized countries, a societal transformation appears to be occurring in the delivery of health care. Health-care providers, for example, are moving from the role of medical 'authority' to that of health-care 'facilitator', guiding patients and consumers through a growing body of medical information. This is

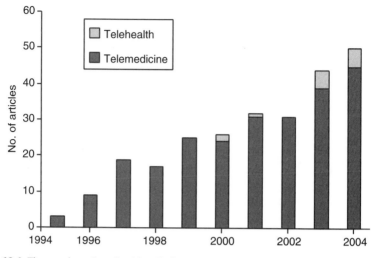

Figure 13.1 The number of studies identified as clinical trials through MEDLINE using the search terms 'telemedicine' and 'telehealth'

one aspect of the move from industrial-age to information-age health-care delivery, and a more patient-centred model of care.[28]

In addition to changes in the roles of patient and provider, social norms are encouraging technology-enabled health care. The Internet and the mobile phone are becoming accepted for everyday transactions such as shopping, banking, voice communication, instant messaging, email and information-seeking. The Internet is already being used to communicate and schedule appointments,[29] and the transition to clinical telemedicine applications seems inevitable.

Although laws regarding medical licensure, malpractice and patient privacy have tended to inhibit the use of telemedicine in the past, supportive regulation is now appearing at the national and state levels. In the USA, for example, the federal government recently appointed a health-care IT coordinator to oversee the integration of communication technologies, including telemedicine.[30]

In contrast, health-care delivery in the developing world remains under-funded, at odds with traditional indigenous practices, physician-centred, and accessible primarily at urban centres and remote health facilities with limited resources. Although Internet and mobile phone use is increasing throughout the developing world, only a fraction of the population use them routinely. The potential impact of international telemedicine is significant.[31,32]

Economic factors

Most health systems in the world are supported through public funding, but many depend heavily on the contribution of the private sector as well. In the USA, health-care costs continue to rise and millions of people remain uninsured. Personnel shortages and decreasing third-party reimbursement are now significant drivers of technology-enabled health care in the industrialized world, particularly in the areas of home care and self-care. This will only intensify as populations age.

Regardless of the source of funding, establishing reimbursement mechanisms for telemedicine remains a challenge. Broad public financing has already resulted in large-scale telemedicine deployment within the health systems of several industrialized countries, including Canada, Australia, New Zealand and the UK, as well as the Veterans Administration (VA) system and statewide networks within the USA. However, demonstrating a return on investment remains critical to the sustainability of telemedicine.

Beyond third-party payers, there has also been growth in the patient-centred consumer health-care market, independent of professional health services. This has led to increased availability of over-the-counter and online diagnostic tests, monitoring devices and medications. Telemedicine services will almost certainly find a niche within this marketplace as well.

Finally, it is unlikely that public health-care funding will be diverted into new delivery mechanisms such as telemedicine in developing countries. In these settings, telemedicine will probably continue to be grant-supported and will therefore continue to face the challenge of economic sustainability. Even low-cost telemedicine will require private sector financing.

Technology

We can safely assume that developments in mobile communications, sensor devices and nanotechnology will alter the way that health care is delivered in the future. Mobile phones and other mobile communication devices will become smaller, less expensive, more powerful, easier to use and will be available at the point of care. Sensors will become more sensitive, passive, wearable and, in some instances, nearly invisible to the user.

Communications infrastructure and services are becoming almost ubiquitous, and there has been substantial uptake of broadband technologies in recent years.[33] Unfortunately, however, a significant 'digital divide' persists among developing countries, limiting future telemedicine services.[32] Figure 13.2 compares the diffusion of communications technologies in the developing world with that of the wealthier countries that form the Organization for Economic Co-operation and Development (OECD). The future challenges to telemedicine are summarized in Box 13.1.

What future applications of telemedicine will emerge?

In general, it is likely that health-care delivery in the industrialized world will continue to move further into the patient's home and to travel with patients wherever they go. The future of monitoring will move from the management of chronic disease to include those recently diagnosed, those predisposed to illness, the 'worried well' and the health conscious. In the not too distant future, this information will also be incorporated into the patient's electronic medical record.

Box 13.1 Challenges for the future of telemedicine

Human factors
Individuals
- Address concerns about training, liability, patient security and increased workload among providers

Organizations
- Demonstrate the value of telemedicine to the health payer, provider and advocacy organizations
- Align telemedicine with the increasing emphasis on self-care and multidisciplinary care models
- Continue clinical trials at academic institutions to demonstrate that telemedicine is effective and efficient

Society
- Promote acceptance of a patient-centred and technology-enabled method of health-care delivery
- Create practice environments that reduce defensive medicine practices, which in turn limit the adoption of new clinical interventions such as telemedicine (e.g. malpractice reform)
- Create a compelling case for lifting licensure restrictions that inhibit telemedicine activities across borders

Economics
- Pilot new third-party reimbursement mechanisms to attract greater patient and provider participation, particularly in health systems that are not supported publicly
- Explore global markets for telemedicine that allow the export of medical expertise
- Seek sustainable economic models that support telemedicine in the developing world to address the growing burden of chronic disease

Technology
- Improve usability for patients with limited function, but who aim to benefit from telemedicine
- Implement methods that verify and authorize access to health information such as fingerprint and voice recognition
- Create communications devices that are smaller, less expensive and more powerful, which will be available at the point of care
- Create sensors that are more sensitive, less expensive, passive and less obtrusive
- Introduce methods of bridging the 'digital divide' faced by developing countries

---

This will also complement multidisciplinary team approaches to care by allowing patients, their carers and providers with varying levels of skill to contribute collectively to the care process.[34]

Advances in mobile and sensor technology will continue to evolve and 'smart' environments will allow passive and invisible monitoring and screening. The mobile phone, for example, will no longer be thought of as simply a device for voice communication, but rather as an access vehicle to multimedia technology, with multiple functions including health-related services. The following scenarios illustrate what telemedicine may look like in the decade ahead.

Patient–provider communication and follow-up care

We are already seeing the gradual adoption of electronic communication between patients and their providers for appointment scheduling, transmission of laboratory results and brief messages.[29] This can be expected to gain momentum as providers become more comfortable with this form of communication. For example, Partners Telemedicine in Boston have a Dermatology e-Visits programme, which allows routine follow-up care for acne patients using the patient's home computer and digital camera. This programme overcomes the long waiting times and travel commonly associated with this type of specialty care.

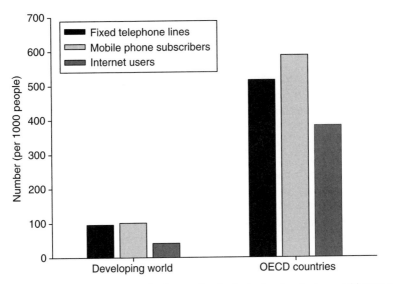

Figure 13.2 The diffusion of communications technologies in the developing world compared with that of the wealthier countries that form the OECD

Disease monitoring and screening

Patient-centred applications that allow greater patient participation from home and facilitate self-care practices are likely to coincide with the increasing availability of easy-to-use, point-of-care diagnostic tests. Diabetic patients in the future, for example, will probably perform not only glucose testing at home, but also risk assessment through haemoglobin A_{1c} measurement and urine microalbumin screening – each of which may become part of accepted self-care practices. Electronic medical records will include the resulting data, which will be widely accessible to all members of the health team who are monitoring and providing care.

Specialist consultations and second opinions

Today, telemedicine is used routinely in specialties such as radiology, pathology, dermatology and psychiatry. We can expect it to become the norm in other areas as well. Cancer patients, for instance, may routinely seek Internet-based second opinions as a way of ensuring that they are doing everything possible to battle their disease. Special populations who face unique obstacles to receiving care, such as prisoners or soldiers, can also expect to receive a greater proportion of their consultative (and monitoring) care via telemedicine in the future.

Intensive and emergency care

The use of telemedicine and telemonitoring in the emergency and critical care of patients is proving not only to be feasible but also effective.[35,36] Patients at the end of life account for substantial health-care spending, and remote patients in need of emergency or intensive care face increased risks associated with transport. Telemedicine will play a larger role in these areas as the clinical and cost benefits become more evident to patients, providers and payers.

Web-based health records including multimedia

When issues of patient privacy are solved, electronic medical records (EMRs) will not only have text and numbers but also other medically relevant data, including still images and videorecordings such as echocardiograms, endoscopies and patient interviews. This will allow specialists, local providers and students located at multiple sites to review archived studies, visualize the course of a patient's disease and obtain a richer educational experience.

Quality assurance and education

Quality assurance and education are intimately linked. Consider a tuberculosis (TB) screening programme in the developing world that allows experienced radiologists to review chest radiographs of suspected TB patients located at distant referral hospitals. This could redistribute expertise, not only for clinical care. It could also be used to assess the performance of local doctors in their ability to read radiographs, and provide them with a unique training opportunity.

Conclusion

The growth and integration of ICTs into health-care delivery holds great potential for patients, providers and payers in health systems of the future. Some answers to the questions about the future of telemedicine are summarized in Table 13.1. Perhaps the most difficult question to answer, however, is 'When will

Table 13.1 Considerations for the future of telemedicine

Question	Issue	Mechanism
Why	Added value	Enable effectiveness, quality, cost-savings and accessibility
Who	Patients/consumers	Healthy, worried well, at-risk, and ill
	Providers	Physicians, nurses, carers and others
	Payers	Public and private
Where	Industrialized world	Patient/consumer's home and body
	Developing world	Traditional health centres and referral hospitals
How	Human factors	Increased adoption among providers and patients/consumers
		Supportive policies, laws and social norms
	Economics	Third-party reimbursement (public and private)
		Entrance into consumer health-care market
	Technology	Small, increasingly passive, affordable, wearable
		Ubiquitous Internet and wireless connectivity
What	Clinical	Screening, diagnostic, monitoring, consulting applications
	Non-clinical	Education and administration applications

telemedicine become part of the standard of care?' Only our actions now will determine the answer to this most difficult question. In the words of a pioneer and visionary in the field of computer science, Alan Kay, 'The best way to predict the future is to invent it'.

References

1   Yellowlees PM, Brooks PM. Health online: the future isn't what it used to be. *Med J Aust* 1999;**171**:522–5
2   Bashshur RL. Where we are in telemedicine/telehealth, and where we go from here. *Telemed J E Health* 2001;**7**:273–7
3   Frey K, Bratton RL. Role of telemedicine in the health care delivery system. *J Am Board Fam Pract* 2002;**15**:170–1
4   Wilson M. The future of telemedicine. *Stud Health Technol Inform* 2002;**80**:129–36
5   Yach D, Hawkes C, Gould CL, Hofman KJ. The global burden of chronic diseases. Overcoming impediments to prevention and control. *JAMA* 2004;**291**:2616–21
6   Organization for Economic Co-Operation and Development (OECD). *Towards High-Performing Health Systems*. Paris: OECD Publishing, 2004
7   Pew Internet and American Life Project. *The Future of the Internet: In a Survey, Technology Experts and Scholars Evaluate Where the Network is Headed in the Next Ten Years*. Washington, DC: Pew Internet, 2005. See http://www.pewinternet.org/pdfs/PIP_Future_of_Internet.pdf (last checked 9 March 2005)
8   Bashshur RL. Telemedicine/telehealth: an international perspective. Telemedicine and health care. *Telemed J E Health* 2002;**8**:5–12
9   Brown SJ. Next generation telecare and its role in primary and community care. *Health Soc Care Commun* 2003;**11**:459–62
10 Meyer M, Kobb R, Ryan P. Virtually healthy: chronic disease management in the home. *Dis Manag* 2002;**5**:87–94
11 Vaccaro J, Cherry J, Harper A, O'Connell M. Utilization reduction, cost savings, and return on investment for PacifiCare Chronic Heart Failure Program, 'Taking Charge of Your Heart Health'. *Dis Manag* 2001;**4**:131–42
12 Bellazzi R, Arcelloni M, Bensa G, *et al*. Design, methods, and evaluation directions of a multi-access service for the management of diabetes mellitus patients. *Diabetes Technol Ther* 2003;**5**:621–9
13 Rogers MA, Small D, Buchan DA, *et al*. Home monitoring service improves mean arterial pressure in patients with essential hypertension. A randomized, controlled trial. *Ann Intern Med* 2001;**134**:1024–32
14 Kobb R, Hoffman N, Lodge R, Kline S. Enhancing elder chronic care through technology and care coordination: report from a pilot. *Telemed J E Health* 2003;**9**:189–95
15 Cherry JC, Moffatt TP, Rodriguez C, Dryden K. Diabetes disease management program for an indigent population empowered by telemedicine technology. *Diabetes Technol Ther* 2002;**4**:783–91
16 Kedar I, Ternullo JL, Weinrib CE, Kelleher KM, Brandling-Bennett H, Kvedar JC. Internet based consultations to transfer knowledge for patients requiring specialised care: retrospective case review. *BMJ* 2003;**326**:696–9
17 Graham LE, Zimmerman M, Vassallo DJ, *et al*. Telemedicine – the way ahead for medicine in the developing world. *Trop Doct* 2003;**33**:36–8
18 Pew Internet and American Life Project. *A Decade of Adoption: How the Internet has Woven Itself into American Life*. Pew Internet and American Life Project, 25 January 2005. See http://207.21.232.103/PPF/r/148/report_display.asp (last checked 23 March 2005)
19 Nesbitt TS, Marcin JP, Daschbach MM, Cole SL. Perceptions of local health care quality in 7 rural communities with telemedicine. *J Rural Health* 2005;**21**:79–85
20 Wood DL. The physician workforce: a medical school dilemma. *Health Aff (Millwood)* 2003;**22**:97–9
21 Spetz J, Given R. The future of the nurse shortage: will wage increases close the gap? *Health Aff (Millwood)* 2003;**22**:199–206
22 Richards H, King G, Reid M, *et al*. Remote working: survey of attitudes to eHealth of doctors and nurses in rural general practices in the United Kingdom. *Fam Pract* 2005;**22**:2–7
23 Hibbert D, Mair FS, May CR, *et al*. Health professionals' responses to the introduction of a home telehealth service. *J Telemed Telecare* 2004;**10**:226–30

24   Porter ME, Teisberg EO. Redefining competition in health care. *Harvard Business Review*, June 2004:64–76

25   Shaller D, Sofaer S, Findlay SD, Hibbard JH, Delbanco S. Consumers and quality-driven health care: a call to action. *Health Aff (Millwood)* 2003;**22**:95–101

26   Strategy 2004–2007: eHealth for Health-care Delivery. World Health Organization, 2004. See http://www.who.int/eht/en/eHealth_HCD.pdf (last checked 9 March 2005)

27   Hailey D, Ohinmaa A, Roine R. Study quality and evidence of benefit in recent assessments of telemedicine. *J Telemed Telecare* 2004;**10**:318–24

28   Smith R. The future of healthcare systems. *BMJ* 1997;**314**:1495–6

29   Liederman EM, Morefield CS. Web messaging: a new tool for patient–physician communication. *J Am Med Inform Assoc* 2003;**10**:260–70

30   US Department of Health and Human Services, Office of the National Coordinator for Health Information Technology (ONCHIT). See http://www.hhs.gov/healthit/framework.html (last checked 9 March 2005)

31   Robinson DF, Savage GT, Campbell KS. Organizational learning, diffusion of innovation, and international collaboration in telemedicine. *Health Care Manage Rev* 2003;**28**:68–78

32   Chandrasekhar CP, Ghosh J. Information and communication technologies and health in low income countries: the potential and the constraints. *Bull World Health Organ* 2001;**79**:850–5

33   National Telecommunications and Information Administration. *A Nation Online: Entering the Broadband Age*. See http://www.ntia.doc.gov/reports/anol/index.html (last checked 23 March 2005)

34   Wiecha J, Pollard T. The interdisciplinary eHealth team: chronic care for the future. *J Med Internet Res* 2004;**6**:e22

35   Breslow MJ, Rosenfeld BA, Doerfler M, *et al.* Effect of a multiple-site intensive care unit telemedicine program on clinical and economic outcomes: an alternative paradigm for intensivist staffing. *Crit Care Med* 2004;**32**:31–8

36   Brebner EM, Brebner JA, Ruddick-Bracken H, *et al.* Evaluation of an accident and emergency teleconsultation service for north-east Scotland. *J Telemed Telecare* 2004;**10**:16–20

►14

Conclusion

Richard Wootton, John Craig and Victor Patterson

There is no doubt that telemedicine works in the right circumstances – works in the sense of being clinically effective and economically efficient. Used correctly, it permits health care to be delivered where previously it was difficult or impossible to do so, and to be improved in situations where there were deficiencies in services. In other circumstances, such as in the exchange of health-care information, it is actually superior to the best traditional methods, allowing easier, more equitable access to information. The 'art' of telemedicine is therefore in being able to choose the appropriate situations in which to make use of it. This book contains the collective experiences of a number of individuals who have, for the most part, identified such situations and in many cases have then gone on to develop successful, and so far sustainable, telemedicine programmes. Common to all their experiences has been the need to start by identifying a deficient or inefficient area of health-care delivery, and then and only then, after traditional alternatives have been exhausted, to consider telemedicine as an option.

Crucial to this process is the need to evaluate the effect of any telemedicine venture properly, and in particular to obtain formal evidence of cost-effectiveness. This is important because without evidence in favour of the cost implication of a telemedicine programme, health-care providers are unlikely to implement such services to a significant degree. This, however, raises questions about how telemedicine research should be funded. Clearly, for telemedicine to develop as a significant means of providing health care, there must be adequate funding for research and evaluation. The potential sources for such funding are many, but public funds should probably be the main source for preliminary phase and pilot projects, with funding for the operational implementation of telemedicine programmes and their evaluation on a large scale coming from private investment for commercial services, or government sources for public health services. As a part of this commitment to providing funding, it is crucial that the developing world, for which the benefits of telemedicine are potentially great (Figure 14.1), should not be forgotten.[1] Continued promotion of telemedicine, by international organizations such as the World Health Organization and others, is a method by which the needs of the developing world might be addressed.[2]

Despite the need for coordinated and strategic planning to fund telemedicine research, potential targets for telemedicine should be chosen pragmatically, and based on a fundamental desire to address the health needs of people and their communities. Who is best placed to identify such targets is debatable, and will vary from one situation to another, but those who have 'hands on' contact

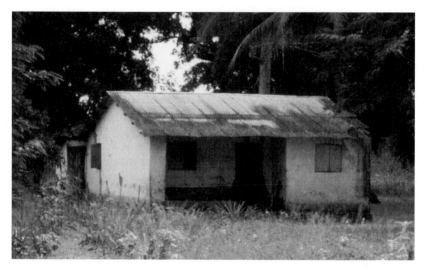

Figure 14.1 Primary health care in an isolated East African village is delivered in a building without electricity or communications. Telemedicine has great potential in these circumstances, although it is likely that only relatively simple forms will be appropriate[3–5] (photo credit: R Wootton).

with the consumers of health care must be included as an integral part of any development process. Providing proper funding for research that is led by the health-care workers themselves is an important step in ensuring that such telemedicine champions are not alienated or marginalized by the establishment.

Indeed, by having health-care workers and consumers as the driving forces of telemedicine, it is more likely that technological developments that have been proceeding at an astonishing pace will begin to take account of the needs of health-care users. This is somewhat in contrast with what has occurred up to now, since most telemedicine equipment represents the offshoots of ventures developed for the business world, whose needs are often very different. If this continues, and health-care workers and users are unable to influence the process of change, the result could be that technology outpaces the abilities of most users to keep up – intellectually, practically or financially. This could result in a relative reduction in the number of people benefiting from technological advances, with an even greater push towards commercialization; in other words, a true shift towards telemedicine being technology and financially driven, and a further shift away from it being driven by health-care needs.

Ensuring that telemedicine programmes are built from the 'bottom up', by individuals or organizations whose primary goal is not one of financial reward, is also more likely to meet another challenge of telemedicine: that systems and programmes should be as simple as possible to meet the health needs of the population of interest. For many telemedicine applications this means that prerecorded systems should be considered before more sophisticated, realtime systems. Technological simplicity will also make acceptance of telemedicine easier within a medical profession that sometimes appears conservative and technophobic. In the 21st century, many doctors still do not use email regularly and even fewer use videoconferencing routinely.

Even so, it should be clear from the material in this book that telemedicine is fundamentally about people and their health needs, rather than about technology and its development, so that human and organizational factors are likely to be the main determinants of how successfully telemedicine can be used. Carefully conducted research has identified the factors that are critical to the success of a telemedicine programme. These include: the need to promote its potential and actual benefits across all cultures, irrespective of social, economic or linguistic barriers; the need to integrate telemedicine within health systems; and the need to address and harmonize legal and regulatory issues between and within countries, and health-care systems.

Telemedicine, like all medicine, is constantly changing and evolving, but the speed with which it has burst onto the medical scene is in contrast to many other aspects of health care, and this may be off-putting to some practitioners. For others, however, this is one of the things that make telemedicine so attractive. As more and more individuals make use of and benefit from telemedicine, and realistically as the technology involved comes to play a greater role in other aspects of our lives, it is hoped that the term 'telemedicine' will no longer be perceived as representing a distinct method for delivering health care. At this time telemedicine will truly have come of age.

References

1   World Health Organization. *A Health Telematics Policy* (document DGO/98.1). Geneva: WHO, 1998
2   Wootton R. The possible use of telemedicine in developing countries. *J Telemed Telecare* 1997;**3**:23–6
3   Martinez A, Villarroel V, Seoane J, del Pozo F. A study of a rural telemedicine system in the Amazon region of Peru. *J Telemed Telecare* 2004;**10**:219–25
4   Lee S, Broderick TJ, Haynes J, Bagwell C, Doarn CR, Merrell RC. The role of low-bandwidth telemedicine in surgical prescreening. *J Pediatr Surg* 2003;**38**:1281–3
5   Wootton R, Youngberry K, Swinfen P, Swinfen R. Prospective case review of a global e-health system for doctors in developing countries. *J Telemed Telecare* 2004;**10** (Suppl. 1):94–6

Index

Page numbers in **bold** indicate figures and tables.